GENETICS
The Nutrition Connection

Ruth M. DeBusk, Ph.D., R.D.

D1568954

AMERICAN
DIETETIC
ASSOCIATION
Chicago, Illinois

Diana Faulhaber, Publisher
Judith Clayton, Managing Editor
Cover design by David Zwierz

10 9 8 7 6 5 4 3 2

Library of Congress Cataloging-in-Publication Data

DeBusk, Ruth M.
  Genetics: the nutrition connection / Ruth M. DeBusk.
    p. ; cm.
Includes bibliographical references and index.
  ISBN 0-88091-195-6
  1. Human genetics. 2. Medical genetics. 3. Nutrition–Genetic aspects.
  [DNLM: 1. Diet Therapy. 2. Genetics, Medical.
  3. Metabolism–genetics. 4. Nutrition.   QZ 50 D289g 2002] I. Title.

QH431 .D344 2002
616'.042–dc21
                              2002013150

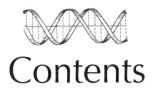

Contents

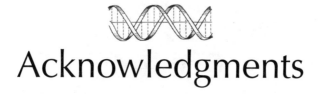

Acknowledgments

This book is dedicated to

My husband, Gib DeBusk, Ph.D., for his stimulating scientific
discussions and never-ending patience during the writing of this book;

My colleagues Bette Bischoff, R.D., C.D.E., and Judy Shabert, M.D., M.P.H., for
their critical reading of the manuscript; to the nutrition
professionals who provided thoughtful peer reviews; and

My editors, Anne Coghill and Diana Faulhaber, who were a joy to work with
and without whose encouragement this book would never have been written.

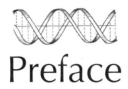

Preface

T his book is for all of us at some level. No one aware of the news today can escape the growing emphasis on genetics in everyday life and the massive investment the world is putting into the multinational Human Genome Project. This book explores how genetics and genetics-based technologies will affect us both as nutrition professionals and as citizens, what the Human Genome Project is and why it promises to revolutionize medical care and nutrition therapy as we know it, applications that are expected to emerge from genetic research in general and the Human Genome Project in particular, and it provides an explanation of fundamental genetic principles so that these applications are readily understandable.

Considerable thought has gone into demystifying genetics and making this book relevant to today's practitioner. Most nutrition professionals have not had the advantage of building a genetics foundation while in school and have had limited opportunities to fill this gap during their busy postgraduate careers, leaving us with no framework on which to hang all the genetics information suddenly bombarding us. The situation is compounded by the unique language and laboratory jargon of the field. Learning genetics on the fly is not a challenge just to nutrition professionals—none of the academic curricula for the health-related professions includes more than a superficial overview. Yet genetics is becoming fundamental in many ways to health maintenance. Consulting genetic profiles in preventive medicine, matching medical therapies to patients' biochemical abilities, selecting drugs that will have the desired effect based on patients' genetic makeup, and matching food to the individual's genetically determined ability to use it in health-beneficial ways will all come from greater understanding of genetics. Clearly, genetics cuts across virtually all health-related disciplines, and health care professionals need to have a working knowledge of basic genetics, of the impact of the Human Genome Project, and of how these basic principles and appliccations apply to health care.

Although it is necessary to learn the basic principles and to be able to speak the language of the field, you will find genetics to be a logical, predictable science once these challenges are mastered. From this base, you can develop a framework on which you can hang new facts as they emerge. It is not necessary to know every detail. What is important and incredibly powerful is to understand the logic of how genetics and its biochemical translation of genes into proteins that perform the work of cells underlies every biochemical reaction that in turn determines every physiological function of every cell in every tissue in the human body. Armed with this insight, practitioners can assemble known, often incomplete facts into useful hypotheses that can guide the development of individualized nutrition therapy.

As our understanding of genetics increases, it will become clear that the present concept of the so-called average person is a myth. Such a person does not exist—individuals are unique in terms of their genetics and therefore in their biochemistry and how they function. Health policy at both the individual and societal levels is based on this myth of the average person. Genetics will have a profound effect on how we approach the development of public health and nutrition policy.

This book is an overview of health- and nutrition-related applications of genetics and the key principles underlying these applications. It is not intended to be the ultimate reference book. Instead, it is intended to be a wake-up call for nutrition professionals and will hopefully stimulate discussion among practitioners, educators, and policy makers about how genetics is forcing changes in our basic concepts of nutrition and what those changes portend for nutrition professionals. New thinking, new tools, and new training will be needed. We have some time before the full impact of genetic advancement is felt; we must use that time wisely to ferret out these needs and address them so that nutrition professionals are positioned to take full advantage of the expanding opportunities that lie ahead.

Genetics is emerging as the central science of medicine. Nutrition will emerge as the central science of *preventive* medicine, and nutrition professionals will play a unique and valuable role in the health care of the future. Be there.

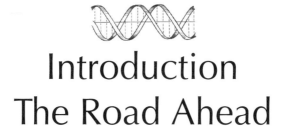

Introduction
The Road Ahead

Genetics would seem to be far removed from nutrition, but actually, we are being exposed to genetics in the news on a daily basis. Just a sampling of recent headlines points out how frequently genetics-related events occur in the news: *Rapist Leaves Genes at Scene; Rough Draft of Human 'Book of Life' Completed; Genetics to Revolutionize Medicine; Serial Killer Nabbed by Genetic Testing; Genetically Engineered Rice May Prevent Vitamin A Deficiency; Scientists Find Protein That Turns Carbs into Fat;* and *Gene Therapy for Boy-in-the-Bubble Disease.* These headlines are of interest to us as citizens certainly but also as nutrition professionals. At the very least, we need to be able to distinguish the credible from the incredible. At most, we need to be able to use genetic information to guide the therapies we recommend to our clients.

GENETICS AND NUTRITION?

Why on earth would a nutrition professional need to know about genetics? Because failure to understand the genetic underpinnings of health and disease can undercut the effectiveness of our nutrition advice. Failure of a dietary plan to support weight loss, decrease LDL-cholesterol levels, or reduce high blood pressure is not necessarily a failure on our part or our client's part: it could be a matter of the wrong plan for the client's genetic makeup. Genetics is now being recognized as the central science of medicine, and it is being integrated into all aspects of health care. Health care professionals are increasingly expected to understand genetics and its influence on health. Additionally, we and our clients are being exposed to news about the results of genetics research on a daily basis.

Genes determine our ability to process food into molecules our cells need and to use these nutrients to support the health of our bodies. Mixing genes in particular combinations through conventional breeding programs is the basis for the development of the edible plant and animal food crops that we depend on for nourishment. Technologies resulting from genetic research are changing the face of agriculture, medical diagnostics and therapy, and pharmacology.

Genetics will similarly change the face of nutrition therapy. Genes are responsible for establishing the limits of our personal health continuum, that is, whether we will be prone to wellness or illness. Until recently we have thought of genetics as sealing our fate: we were stuck with our genes, and we came to admire people who accepted their fate and gracefully played the genetic hands they were dealt. Much of our medical, societal, and educational orientation has focused on compensating for our various genetic limitations.

The new and truly wonderful discovery is that genetics does not necessarily determine our destiny—it only sets the upper and lower limits of our functional ability. More exciting still is the realization that nutrition is a major factor in modifying the messages our genes contain. As we come to better understand the interrelationships among genes and external influences such as nutrition and other lifestyle choices (what we call our environment), nutrition professionals will have at their disposal an awesome set of tools with which to tailor nutrition therapy to the desired genetic outcomes.

Why Now?

Genetics has grabbed the spotlight as the result of the Human Genome Project, a worldwide collaborative effort to understand everything imaginable about human genetic information, including how genes lead to disease and how we can intervene to head off that outcome. The reach of genetics will be felt well beyond the linkage of a single gene to a particular disease, however. Genetics is evolving into genomics, a field that involves identifying each building block of the genetic material, each protein whose synthesis is directed by that genetic material, what these proteins do in reference to the work of the cells, how the synthesis of these proteins is turned on and off in response to environmental signals, and how genes interact with each other. Genomics is a global view of how we and other organisms function, both within our internal environment and within the larger environment around us.

As these mysteries unfold, the promise of genomics includes ever-increasingly sophisticated technologies that allow genetic manipulation of feed crops and animals, genetics-based diagnostic tests that allow determination of which disorders an individual is at risk for developing, to which drugs an individual will react positively or negatively, and which foods a person will process effectively and beneficially. This type of information lays the foundation for a coming era of medical and nutritional therapy that is personalized for each individual's genetic uniqueness.

With this progress will come tough decisions as to how we as a society handle this information and the powerful capabilities that result. How will we protect the privacy of the genetic information of our citizens? How will we ensure that the information is used fairly and not to discriminate against an individual? How will access to gene testing and gene therapy be determined? How will we ensure that food developed with genetic technology is safe?

If personalized health care is the wave of the future, how will we educate our health care professionals and those who teach them? If genetics will have such a pervasive impact on our society, how will we educate our citizens so that informed choices can be made? How will we develop public health policy that moves away from a one-size-fits-all approach and integrates the need to address the genetic uniqueness of every citizen?

This book will explore many issues to provide you with an overview of how genetics will affect us as health care professionals and as private citizens. We will look first at the Human Genome Project, which more than any other event is responsible for catapulting human genetics light-years ahead in terms of applications to health. Next we will fill in just enough background genetics to make sense of all the applications that are coming, many of which will be discussed in this book. Then we will tackle the tough questions of the implications of genetic research on society, in terms of the ethical, social, and legal implications, and on food and nutrition policy. Finally, we will discuss opportunities for the nutrition professional within this genetics revolution.

Is there a place for the nutrition professional in these exciting developments? You bet! Front and center. Nutrition will turn out to be a powerful–possibly the *most* powerful–means of modifying the messages in our genes.

1

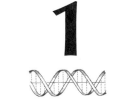

Genomics:
The New Genetics

The terms *genetics* and *genomics* appear in the news frequently, and they are often used interchangeably, much to the confusion of the reader at times. The same goes for "new" and "old" genetics. We are observing a field in transition, in which the focus, the tools, and the terminology are all evolving.

GENETICS VERSUS GENOMICS

The term *genetics* connotes a field concerned with single genes that cause distinct traits, whether the subject is people and diseases, or plants and their particular characteristics. *Genomics*, in contrast, gives us a broader view of genetics, and it is often referred to as the "new" genetics. Until just recently genetics focused on breeding programs that improved our ability to feed the global population, both in terms of quantity and quality of plants and livestock, and on dealing with the negative impact that genetics can have on the population's health. Genomics moves beyond single genes and addresses more complex situations in which multiple genes are involved in the development of a disease, and environmental signals can affect the expression of these genes. Also, tools are now available that help us to act rather than to react, to focus on preventive health by understanding an individual's genetic risks and intervening before a disease can manifest.

The vision, goals, and technologies of the so-called new genetics are more sophisticated than those of the old genetics. However, the underlying desire to understand how genetic information is encoded and translated, how its expression is regulated, and how this knowledge can be harnessed to improve food production and health care for people and animals are essentially the same. Genomics is simply the next step in the evolution of our understanding of genetics.

Genetic terminology is in transition. Genetics may come to mean the narrower connotation and genomics the broader one but, for now, many professionals and lay people alike seem reluctant to abandon the term "genetics" as one that encompasses the full spectrum of genetics/genomics. For this book, we will use *genetics* to refer to all aspects of gene-related information, applications, and technology. In general, genetics refers today to the era ahead in which the advances in genetics will have far-reaching effects on food and health for the global population.

The evolution of the concept of genetic information can be seen by tracing the development of the study of genetics, beginning with the Austrian monk Gregor Mendel and continuing through to the Human Genome Project of today, with its ever-broadening goal of a complete understanding of DNA and protein and their impact on health.

THE MENDELIAN VIEW

Gregor Mendel discovered the basic laws of inheritance. He found that a distinctive physical characteristic was inherited in an orderly, predictable manner. Mendel was soon able to predict when a trait would disappear and when it would reappear in subsequent generations, thereby providing us with an understanding of why we had particular genetic limitations and how we passed them on to our children and grandchildren. Mendelian genetics became the science of inheritance, based on straightforward, reproducible, predictable patterns such as blue eyes or being tall. It was subsequently discovered that discrete physical units called chromosomes could be correlated with these orderly inherited patterns, and the mechanics of the inheritance of these chromosomes was elegantly worked out in the first half of the twentieth century.

THE MOLECULAR VIEW

By the 1950s, however, scientists had become intrigued with the makeup of chromosomes and how they carried information from generation to generation. From the work of several contributors, it was discovered that the genetic material contained in the chromosomes was deoxyribonucleic acid (DNA). DNA is a linear molecule made up of four different nitrogenous bases linked one to another; the linear sequence of bases encodes the genetic information. In 1953 James Watson and Francis Crick, building on the work of Rosalind Franklin and other distinguished scientists, deduced the structure of DNA and with it essential information on how the genetic material was able to be faithfully copied and transmitted to each new cell.

Genetic research then shifted to the details of the chemical makeup of chromosomes and understanding the processes by which information was stored in DNA and retrieved in an orderly fashion, as well as how the information was useful to the cells of the organism. The one gene–one protein concept emerged, whereby the genetic information in particular regions of the DNA, called genes, was decoded into a message that was then translated into a protein; such proteins perform the work of the cells. It was clear that a single gene in different people could result in variations on a single trait and that these variations were due to changes in DNA. Such changes in DNA could also result in changes in function; some of these changes were seriously debilitating and even deadly. Among the classic examples of how a single change involving just one of the bases in DNA could result in a serious disorder are sickle cell disease and cystic fibrosis. In both cases a single base change leads to the translation of genetic information into faulty proteins that no longer function normally and have serious consequences to those with these conditions.

At this point genes were studied one at a time by individual scientists. Specifically, the scientists sought to discover on which chromosome the gene for a trait or disorder was located and exactly where on that chromosome it was. The approach was piecemeal: each research team looked at their gene of interest and struggled to figure out how it differed among individuals and to identify its biochemical and physiological effects on function. In an approach similar in concept to what Mendelian geneticists sought to accomplish by looking at large numbers of inheritance patterns, geneticists in the molecular era looked at single genes at a detailed DNA level, connecting changes to physical results.

THE GENOMIC VIEW

The molecular view tended to favor an all-or-none theory in terms of the effect of a change in the DNA on gene function, not that of so-called gene dosing, a graduated effect that corresponded to particular molecular changes. This latter orientation would await the dawn of the genomics era. As geneticists grew more sophisticated in understanding inheritance, they began to realize that not all traits were inherited and expressed in a simple, straightforward way—that there could be a number of genes and influences on those genes contributing to a "characteristic" such as a disease. Mendelian genetics showed that this characteristic was inherited, but the mechanism and the players involved were poorly understood.

At this point, a few of the scientists struggling with the one gene–one protein concept realized that many characteristics such as intelligence, behavior, and chronic diseases involved multiple genes and multiple influences that were somehow communicated from the environment to the genetic material. Their challenge of identifying those genes and influences, as well as understanding just how these factors actually communicated to the genes, amounted to looking for a needle in a haystack. The more visionary among the geneticists realized that there were far too many gaps in fundamental knowledge about human genetic material and its workings and that genetic research needed to move from the traditional, isolated effort to a massive team effort, the likes of which had never before been attempted. Essentially they needed this type of co-operative effort and comprehensive information for *all* of the human genetic material, collectively called the *genome*, essentially an encyclopedia of the human being—a "Book of Life," as it has come to be called.

Their vision became the Human Genome Project. Such a far-reaching effort was only possible, however, because the technology for determining the sequence of the DNA and for manipulating genes was finally available. Although they were crude, at least the basic tools were in place. Molecular geneticists divided the work. One research team took one chromosome; another team took another. Ultimately, the teams would assemble the results into a cohesive whole, a detailed map of the human genome and an understanding of each gene's function.

THE DECADE AHEAD

This brief historical summary brings us to the present day. At this point, we have two key sets of information: the Mendelian map, which tells us where on a particular chromosome a definable trait is located, and the equivalent of a map at the molecular level, which fine-tunes the gross chromosomal map and adds details of the DNA base composition of the chromosomes. It is now possible to begin the monumental task of matching these two by correlating the Mendelian expression of a gene with a particular altered DNA sequence.

Huge gaps in understanding still exist, particularly in terms of the function of the majority of the DNA in the human being and in terms of understanding how genes interact with each other and with influences outside the body, such as nutrients. Present data indicate that there are differences among individuals, but we have little idea what these differences are at the DNA level and how they lead to differences in function. This whole puzzle is the study of *proteomics*–the identification of the protein products that result from expressing the genes, and the elaboration of their function in the organism. Essentially the plan is to do at the protein level what the Human Genome Project is doing at the DNA level.

Knowledge of how genes work, and their role in health and disease, is already being applied to medicine and pharmacology. As our understanding of nutritional effects on genetic outcomes grows, nutrition therapy will similarly become gene-directed in an emerging field called *nutritional genomics.* Nutrients, whether from food or from supplements, are effective in at least three important ways in terms of modifying genetic outcomes. First, they can fill in the biochemical gaps caused by the limitations in our genetic material. Second, they can activate the expression of necessary genetic information to make more of a desirable protein available to cells. Finally, they can also deactivate the expression of genetic information that has a detrimental effect on the organism's function. Genetics-savvy nutrition professionals will be able to use this basic framework to treat clients as unique genetic individuals and tailor their food and supplement intakes to maximize their unique genetic potentials. Using genetics to direct nutrition therapy will emerge as one of the most sophisticated and effective tools ever available to the nutrition professional.

THE GENETICS REVOLUTION'S IMPACT ON NUTRITION

Shifting to genetics-oriented nutrition practice will require a solid understanding of the following:

- Basic genetic principles
- Genetic technologies used for research, food production, and health care diagnostics
- The implications of genetics for medical therapy
- The implications of genetics for nutrition therapy
- The ethical, legal, and social implications of genetics
- The implications of genetics for nutrition policy
- The role of the nutrition professional in a genetics-oriented era of health care

There is no doubt that genetics is having a major impact on food, nutrition, and medicine as we know it and that genetics will be a central science in the era ahead. This paradigm shift will be accompanied by the loss of many traditional roles for nutrition professionals and the emergence of new, more intellectually challenging and outcome-enhancing opportunities for the genetics-savvy nutrition professional. Each of these topics will be explored in the chapters that follow.

Useful Resources

The human genome. *Nature*. 2001; 409 (theme issue):745–964.
The human genome. *Science*. 2001; 291 (theme issue):1145–1434.
Strohman RC. Genomics and human life span—what's left to extend? *Nat Biotechnol*. 2001; 19:195–216.

Useful Web Sites

Basic Genetics/Genomics page. National Institutes of Health Division of Intramural Research's Office of Science Education and Outreach Web site. Available at: http://www.nhgri.nih.gov/DIR/VIP. Accessed July 30, 2002.
Genetics and Genomics on the Web page. National Institutes of Health Web site. Available at: http://www.nhgri.nih.gov/Data. Accessed July 30, 2002.

2

The Human Genome Project

The Human Genome Project has been likened to the dream of putting a man on the moon. No less ambitious, the Human Genome Project's goal of producing the "Book of Life" will provide us with information that will revolutionize medicine. Understanding the direct link between our genetic information and our risk for disease will have profound implications for diagnostics, preventive medicine, and therapeutics.

Medicine will move from a medical surveillance orientation to a therapeutic and preventive orientation. Therapies will be targeted to the biochemistry underlying each human function and the dysfunction that results in disease. Genetic knowledge will enable risk identification and early intervention to prevent development of disease. The great promise of the Human Genome Project is that of personalized medicine, a new approach to health care in which each individual's unique genetic potential can be optimized through appropriate preventive and therapeutic measures.

WHAT IS THE HUMAN GENOME PROJECT?

As explained in Chapter 1, the genome for an organism is its complete set of genetic information. The overall goal of the Human Genome Project is to generate detailed information about the structure, organization, and function of the human genetic material and how it is translated into instructions that guide the development and functioning of the human body. The specific goals have evolved as the project has progressed. Several organisms used as model systems in the research laboratory, from bacteria to mice, are also being studied.

From the beginning the goals have been to identify each nucleotide building block of DNA (commonly referred to as a *DNA base* or simply *base*) in its correct sequence in the human set of genetic information, to figure out which sequences of bases represent genes, and to locate each gene's physical position on a chromosome.

The sequence of bases is the key to the information contained within the genome. The details of DNA as the genetic information, and how that information is translated into useful products and services for each cell, will be discussed in the next chapter. It appears that the vast majority of DNA in a cell does not, at this point in our understanding, appear to be translated into useful products. Those sections of DNA that are translated are called genes. Because there is so much DNA in the nucleus of a human cell, it's not stored as a long linear molecule but instead is broken up into manageable packaging units, called chromosomes. Each gene has a location on a particular chromosome, just as a town has a specific location on a map. The Human Genome Project aims to construct a detailed map of the human genome: all of the genes on all of the chromosomes and every base in between these genes.

Progress on the Human Genome Project has exceeded expectations, and the most recent goals move beyond just describing the genome and now include defining the function of each gene and possibly of the non-gene segments as well. For those bases that form a gene, genome scientists are investigating the details of how that gene's expression is switched on and off, which environmental signals influence gene expression, and how a gene relates to disease.

WHAT ARE THE SPECIFIC GOALS OF THE HUMAN GENOME PROJECT?

Because progress on the project has proceeded at a faster pace than expected, the specific goals have changed over the past decade since the initiation of the project. The original research plan was for the first five years of the fifteen-year project, from 1990 to 1995, and it focused on building an infrastructure of information and on developing the technologies that would enable large-scale cataloging of the various parts of the genome. The specific goals included determining all of the DNA bases, in order, within the human DNA; identifying all of the genes within this sequence of bases; storing the information in databases; developing technologies that permitted fast, efficient sequencing and computer handling of the massive amount of data that would be generated; and addressing the ethical, legal, and social implications of genomic research. Although these were considered extremely ambitious goals that were expected to take the full fifteen years to realize, progress surpassed even the most optimistic projections. As a result, in 1993 a new plan was developed to guide the project through 1998. Focus was still on building the infrastructure and the tools needed, but the vision expanded as it became apparent that a much greater extent of detail would be possible than originally anticipated, so a complete sequence for the human genome, and possibly for several animals, plants, and microorganisms, was well within the scope of the project.

Progress under the second plan was rapid, and a new five-year plan was established for 1998 to 2003. The vision now is to move beyond gathering information to integrating that information into understanding how the component parts of the human genome interact with each other and the environment—a goal that will challenge biological scientists for many decades to come. The work plan for 1998 through 2003 focuses on eight major goals:

- Completing the working draft of the full sequence of the human genome by the end of 2001 (a goal reached in June 2000), completing the full sequence by the end of 2003, and making that sequence freely available to all who want to use it
- Developing sequencing technology to support this effort
- Studying the natural genetic variation among individuals (that is, sequence variation)
- Developing the technology needed to support functional genomics, the scientific discipline concerned with identifying the genes within the genome and studying the function of their gene products
- Continuing to sequence the genomes of several organisms that are used in research laboratories as model systems
- Studying the ethical, legal, and social implications of genome research
- Developing the fields of bioinformatics and computational biology
- Training genome scientists

Specifics of each of these goals follow.

The Human DNA Sequence

The overall goal is to construct a detailed genetic and physical map of the human genome. This effort involves identifying each base in human DNA; dividing those bases into genes, which are functional regions that are translated into proteins that do the work of the cells; and creating a genetic map by physically locating each gene to a particular chromosome and, further, to a specific location on that chromosome. To provide a complete and accurate sequence, readily available to all, is the highest priority of the Human Genome Project. The agreed-upon standard for the finished sequence is no more than a single error for every ten thousand bases. The human sequence is considered a precious scientific resource. Making it accessible to those who can make use of it provides much-needed infrastructure for research scientists and saves considerably in research time and costs.

Sequencing Technology

The project planners also foresaw the need to develop new technologies and to improve existing technologies to support the goals of the project. Before the Human Genome Project, scientists studied one gene and its product at a time. The study of genetics has now shifted to the whole genome, which calls for a different scale of operation in which all of a cell's genes or their protein products can potentially be studied at one time. Among the expected technological outcomes are the following:

- Improved sequencing technology that enables automating this labor-intensive process and that improves the efficiency, accuracy, and cost-effectiveness of the sequencing process
- Technologies that enable the sequencing information to be used to study the natural sequence variation within the human population and its relation to human disease
- The development of functional genomics, a new area of biology that focuses on investigating the function of DNA sequences within the genome and their interaction with the environment
- The ability to compare genomes from a variety of organisms in order to understand fundamental biological mechanisms and the details of gene structure and function
- The development of bioinformatics and computational biology, which are concerned with collecting, analyzing, detailing, and storing the large amounts of data generated by the project, con-

verting the data into user-friendly databases accessible to the public, and enabling scientists to communicate genetic information to each other and to medical personnel

Human Genome Sequence Variation

DNA sequence variation is the raw material of evolution. Having in hand the human genome sequence and those of various other vertebrate organisms enables comparisons among organisms and helps us to understand how human beings evolved. Sequence variation is also the basis for individual uniqueness, including our differences in disease susceptibility and responses to environmental toxins, drugs, foods, and such. Understanding how genetic variation results in these highly individual responses is expected to have a significant impact on how we approach disease prevention and treatment.

A gene with two or more variants that occur in more than one percent of the population is said to be *polymorphic.* Basic information about the types, number, and location of polymorphisms within the human genome is needed. The most common type appears to be the single-nucleotide polymorphism (SNP, pronounced "snip"), in which two genetic sequences are identical except for a single nucleotide (base). SNPs occur about every one hundred to two hundred bases along the DNA sequence (see the article by Stephens et al., listed in the "Useful Resources" section at the end of this chapter). A gene and its associated sequences may have more than one SNP. SNPs are expected to play a major role in predicting individual differences in drug responses and in analyzing the causes of complex disorders such as cancer, diabetes, cardiovascular disease, and mental illness.

Technology for Functional Genomics

Sequencing the human genome is just the first step. The next step is to understand the product of each gene and how that product affects human function. Functional genomics is the scientific discipline concerned with the interpretation of the function of a DNA sequence, which involves the interaction of the genome and its environment. Scientists are particularly interested in linking specific gene sequences with specific diseases. For them to be able to do so, there must first be large-scale characterization of the proteins expressed by each gene. In addition, there are numerous sequences within the genome that do not code for proteins. Some of these sequences serve as regulatory regions that control the expression of the genes. The function of other sequences is unknown. The ultimate goal of functional genomics is to identify the function, if any, of each sequence, whether or not it codes for a protein.

Comparative Genomics: Sequencing of Model Organisms

Genetic research has relied heavily on the development of *model organisms* or *model systems*. Such systems are organisms (animal, plant, or microorganism) that can be readily housed in the laboratory and whose genetics, biochemistry, and physiology can be exhaustively studied. The value of such work lies in the fact that all organisms are related through a common evolutionary tree, so studying one organism can provide insight into other organisms. This approach has been particularly fruitful in molecular genetics, where a number of organisms that can be manipulated genetically and nutritionally have been used to produce meaningful information about the workings of those organisms and, by extrapolation, to more complicated organisms such as human beings. Models from bacteria to the laboratory mouse have provided tremendous insight into how things work in the biology of living systems. In many cases a mouse model, for example, has been developed that mimics a human disease system. The disease process can be studied in the laboratory, suspected key genes can be identified and changes introduced, and the impact of those changes on the disease process can then be determined. Such studies have been invaluable for providing insight into human diseases.

By introducing a mutation into the genetic material of an organism, observing the effect on the organism, and then identifying the gene that has been altered, researchers can deduce quite a bit about the genetic control of a particular function of that organism. Further, model organisms contain many of the same "housekeeping" genes as human beings, so extrapolations can be made from the model organism to human beings. A housekeeping gene is one that is involved with the essential activities that take place at the cellular level, such as energy production or nutrient synthesis.

Studying the genes of model organisms can often serve as a shortcut to understanding human disease. Colorectal cancer is an example. Researchers first found genes in yeast and bacteria that help to repair mistakes that occur during DNA duplication–a kind of "spellchecker" system for detecting and eliminating DNA "typos." By searching genetic databases, these genes were also found in human beings. It was subsequently found that when these repair enzymes were mutated, individuals had a high risk of developing colon cancer.

Initially five model organisms were chosen: the bacterium *Escherichia coli*, the yeast *Saccharomyces cerevisiae*, the parasitic roundworm *Caenorhabditis elegans*, the fruit fly *Drosophila melanogaster*, and the laboratory mouse *Mus musculus*. By now, much of this work has been completed. Many laboratories are participating and contributing sequencing information from a wide variety of model systems, including numerous species of bacteria, the soil-dwelling amoeba *Dictyostelium discoideum*, the roundworm *Caenorhabditis briggsae*, the plant *Arabidopsis thaliana*, the zebrafish *Danio rerio*, the frogs *Xenopus laevis* and *Xenopus tropicalis*, and various strains of the laboratory rat. Additional plant genomes have also been sequenced.

Ethical, Legal, and Social Issues (ELSI)

From the earliest planning stages of the Human Genome Project, the potential ethical, legal, and social implications of the information that was likely to come out of the project have been of concern. A partnership of biological scientists, social scientists, health care professionals, legal scholars, historians, theologians, and others are exploring these issues. As a result, a body of knowledge now exists that can be used to educate the public and to guide genetics research and genetics-related public policy. ELSI research focuses on four major areas of concern:

- Privacy and fair use of genetic information–the need to protect the individual's privacy with respect to the use and interpretation of his or her genetic information and to prevent discrimination based on an individual's genetic information
- Integration of genetic technologies into the clinic–how best to integrate new genetic technologies into clinical practice and ensure adequate informed consent for participants in genetic research
- Ethical issues surrounding genetic research–which issues society will need to address concerning the use of these powerful new technologies
- Professional public education–the need to educate students, health care professionals, policy makers, and the public on the ethical, legal, and social implications of genetic research

The major ELSI concerns are discussed in detail in Chapter 7.

Developing the Fields of Bioinformatics and Computational Biology

Bioinformatics concerns collecting, analyzing, detailing, and storing the huge amount of data being generated by the Human Genome Project. Vast computational, statistical, and applied mathematical support is needed to understand biology in the twenty-first century. In addition to the mechanics of handling this massive amount of data, scientists need to be able to extract information from the databases, view it using graphical displays, analyze it efficiently while comparing human genomic information with that of multiple other organisms, and readily share their findings with others. Computer science is at the heart of this requirement, and part of the focus of the Human Genome Project is to develop bioinformatics and the computational tools needed to handle the data being generated.

A practical application of bioinformatics is for a researcher to enter a newly discovered DNA sequence into the computer and search gene databases to determine whether that sequence is part of a gene that has already been sequenced from another organism. If it is, the researcher immediately has available the information that other researchers have compiled for that gene in other organisms. If no matches to known genes are found, the computer can check whether the sequence is an unknown gene (as opposed to a nongene sequence) by determining whether it has the standard "punctuation" and format characteristics of a gene. If it does, the next step for researchers is to figure out that gene's function. This approach was used to identify the gene for the disease adrenoleukodystrophy, a rare condition now more widely recognized because of the movie *Lorenzo's Oil.* Researchers had not been able to locate the gene for this disease through conventional linkage analysis, but the computer was able to predict the sequence. DNA probes were then constructed that could bind to the gene, and eventually the gene and its chromosomal location were discovered.

Training Genomic Scientists

Historically, biology has benefited from the participation of scientists from disciplines outside biology. As the demand for genomic research grows, there is a particular need to train scientists who can work at the interface of biology and other disciplines, such as computer science, chemistry, mathematics, physics, and the social sciences. Particular shortages include scholars trained in bioinformatics, researchers who can probe the societal impact of genetic discoveries, and scientists with the management skills to lead large data-production operations. A significant contribution of the Human Genome Project will be to ensure an adequate supply of appropriately trained scientists.

WHAT ARE THE EXPECTED INITIAL APPLICATIONS OF THE HUMAN GENOME PROJECT?

Great things are expected to come from the Human Genome Project. Overall the emphasis will shift from genetic (that is, the study of a single gene and its link to disease) to genomic (that is, the impact of multiple genes and their interaction with each other and the environment). Obviously, many applications must await further understanding of the basic science, but some near-term applications look quite promising. Among them are diagnostic testing for DNA sequences that predispose to disease, pharmacological applications such as targeted drug therapy and drug design, and customized nutrition therapy.

Diagnostic Testing

Once a DNA sequence has been positively identified as being linked to increased susceptibility to a medical condition, a genetic diagnostic test can be developed. To be a useful test, though, the sequence when detected must indicate with near 100 percent reliability the presence of the gene that predisposes to the condition of interest. DNA diagnostic tests are already available for sickle cell disease, hemochromatosis, cystic fibrosis, familial hypercholesterolemia, Huntington's disease, and osteogenesis imperfecta, to name just a few. The details of genetic testing and the ethical, legal, and social implications of such testing will be discussed in later chapters.

Pharmacogenomics

The ability to use genetic information to design drugs that specifically target a susceptible protein or to classify a population into those who will respond to a particular drug and thereby benefit from its use, those who will not benefit, those who will experience side effects (possibly toxic), and those who will neither benefit nor be harmed, is a new discipline called *pharmacogenomics,* a marriage of pharmacology with genomics.

One gene family that exists in a multitude of variations generates cytochrome P450 (CYP 450), an enzyme system found in the liver and in the lining of the small intestine. Several different genes make up this family, and each gene has multiple variations. If we took just one of the genes that codes for a particular CYP 450 enzyme and compared this enzyme among a large number of people, we would find a great deal of variation in terms of the functioning of the enzyme. Some people would have a high level of function, some medium, some low, and some none at all. If we gave each of these individuals a drug that required this particular CYP 450 to metabolize it before it could be useful to the body, the response to the drug would fall into the same four categories: excellent conversion (maybe even making too much of the drug available for absorption into the body and causing an overdose); a normal level of conversion, so that the drug gave these individuals the expected therapeutic effect; poor conversion, so that these individuals were underserved by the drug; and no conversion at all, which would mean these individuals would not benefit from the drug. With all this variation for a single drug, it should be clear from this discussion that drugs need to be matched to the genetic constitution of each individual. Such matching is on the horizon thanks to the Human Genome Project. A more detailed treatment of predicting an individual's response to a drug prior to its being taken is given in Chapter 5.

Once the product of a disease susceptibility gene is known, drugs can be developed that specifically target a vulnerable spot in that protein or might target the control region that regulates the expression of the gene itself. The technology to perform computer modeling of such targets exists; what is needed now is information about the gene and its protein product. The Human Genome Project will supply just such information.

Customized Nutrition Therapy (Nutritional Genomics)

Initial emphasis in personalizing nutrition therapy will be on single genes that result in disease. The sheer complexity of multiple genes and multiple environmental influences makes it common sense to work first with the more straightforward, but still complex, situation of a single gene and its product and how they lead to a disorder. Nutrition can have a variety of effects. The gene may result in a biochemical limitation—perhaps the protein coded for by the gene is not fully functional, resulting in less of a metabolite being generated than the cell requires. In such a situation, nutrition, whether as food or as supplements, can supply the missing compound. There are already numerous examples of this use of nutrition therapy, such as supplying vitamin C every day to compensate for our inability to make the enzyme gulonolactone oxidase or ensuring adequate intake of the amino acid tyrosine to compensate for the lack of phenylalanine hydroxylase in persons with phenylketonuria. A faulty enzyme may cause harmful intermediates in the metabolic pathway to accumulate; for example, elevated levels of homocysteine increase the risk of heart disease. Nutrition therapy with the B vitamins folic acid, vitamin B-12, and vitamin B-6 focuses on ways to convert homocysteine to less harmful metabolites.

Nutrition can also work at the level of the control of gene expression. Perhaps a disorder in which too much of a compound accumulates is due not to a faulty enzyme but to too much production of that enzyme. Through nutrition, compounds can be supplied that may reduce the expression of the gene and thus the synthesis of its enzyme product, resulting in a lesser amount of that compound being made. Alternatively, nutrition may increase gene expression. Rather than decreasing the production of an enzyme that produces toxic levels of a compound, another approach is to use nutrition to increase the expression of another gene whose enzyme product can take the toxic compound and convert it to a harmless one. A different example of the benefits of increasing gene expression is to increase the synthesis of an enzyme that generates a metabolite that is beneficial to the cell when present in greater than usual quantities. Here our knowledge is much more elementary than it is with understanding biochemical pathways and how to use nutrition to circumvent limitations to those pathways caused by our genes. Studies are under way to examine how specific nutrients influence gene expression: for one, limonene from citrus and glucosinolates from cruciferous vegetables and their ability to increase the expression of glutathione S-transferase, an important antioxidant defense enzyme; for another, the ability of bioflavonoids such as curcumin and quercetin to decrease pro-inflammatory cytokine production.

HOW WELL IS THE PROJECT MEETING ITS GOALS?

The original goal of the Human Genome Project, to sequence the human genome completely, is now slated to be finished in 2003, which is the fifty-year anniversary of the discovery of the double helical structure of DNA and a fitting tribute to this momentous event in the history of biology. Much can be gained in the shorter term, however, by the construction of a working draft of the genome. The completion of such a rough draft by the combined efforts of the public consortium, overseen by the U.S. Department of Energy and National Institutes of Health and a private sector laboratory, Celera Genomics, was announced at a White House press conference in June 2000. With 97 percent of the human genome sequenced, the major landmarks are in place, but many of the details remain to be discovered, and numerous errors are contained in this first draft. Instead of the 100,000 to 120,000 genes predicted, only approximately 30,000 (estimated at 26,000 to 40,000) could be detected.

Although the draft sequence has gaps and errors, it can be used to find genes that are the focus of numerous current scientific projects, which promise to yield results with considerable time and cost savings. The rough draft now needs to be converted to a finished manuscript. The sequencing needs to be completed, and the public and private sector sequences need to be reconciled. The errors must be resolved, because a high-quality sequence (with no more than a single error every ten thousand bases) is considered essential for recognizing the regulatory components of genes–those sequences critical to a gene's expression. The current work plan for the Human Genome Project calls for completion of the finished sequence by the end of 2003. Like the other goals for the project, this one, too, is proceeding well ahead of schedule.

WHERE IS THE WORK ACTUALLY BEING DONE?

This ambitious project was first conceived within the U.S. Department of Energy in the mid 1980s. The project was formally initiated in 1990 as a fifteen-year multinational collaboration to sequence (that is, to determine, in order, each nucleotide base in) the entire human genome. The project is administered by the United States through the joint efforts of the Office of Biological and Environmental Research of the Life Sciences Division of Oak Ridge National Laboratory, within the U.S. Department of Energy (DOE), and of the National Human Genome Research Institute, within the National Institutes of Health (NIH). Numerous research institutions and universities worldwide are directly involved in the project. In addition, several countries have contributed to the funding of the project. Five sites have been designated as primary Human Genome Project sequencing centers: the Sanger Centre (Hinxton, England); the DOE Joint Genome Project (Walnut Creek, California), which is a collaboration of the Lawrence Livermore, Lawrence Berkeley, and Los Alamos National Laboratories; Baylor College of Medicine (Houston, Texas); Washington University School of Medicine (St. Louis, Missouri); and the Whitehead Institute/MIT Center for Genome Research (Cambridge, Massachusetts). In addition, Celera

Genomics (Rockville, Maryland), a private-sector company headed by J. Craig Venter, Ph.D., mentioned earlier, is also working to sequence the human genome. A nonprofit private-sector venture, the Institute for Systems Biology (Seattle, Washington), headed by Leroy Hood, Ph.D., is focusing on integrating the information into an understanding of how the whole organism works.

WHOSE DNA IS BEING USED?

Although all human beings have the same basic genetic setup, in that we have the same genes in the same chromosomal locations that carry out the same basic functions, each of us has a slightly different base sequence within those genes, which is what gives us our individual uniqueness. No one genome would be precisely representative of all other human beings. Whose genome should be chosen to sequence, then? The decision was made to use the genomes of several individuals, both male and female, from diverse racial and ethnic backgrounds. Considerable care was taken to establish a protocol whereby investigators could not link the genome data with particular individuals and those who donated their DNA could not make direct correlations between the findings of the project and their personal DNA.

WHAT'S NEXT AFTER THE GENOME IS SEQUENCED?

Generating the rough draft of the human genome sequence was the end of the beginning. Whereas it was once the end point of the project, the rapid progress and extent of collaboration make it possible to move beyond just gathering information to understanding how these sequences direct the activities of the cells and how they relate to disease. The next phase is focusing on annotating the genome: locating the genes, determining their gene products and the function of each product, and investigating how gene expression is turned on and off and how the environment influences expression. A number of interesting questions are being addressed. For example, how can only thirty thousand genes be sufficient to code for the complexity of the human being when the roundworm and fruit fly, lower life forms in the biological hierarchy, have nineteen thousand and thirteen thousand genes, respectively? We certainly expected the highly evolved human being to have many times more genes than these much simpler organisms. What are race and ethnicity in the face of the estimate that human beings are 99.9 percent identical in terms of DNA sequence? What are the connections between disease and specific genes and environmental signals? This expansion of the original goals of the project promises to yield exciting results and, quite possibly, more questions than answers.

WHAT CAN WE EXPECT FROM THE HUMAN GENOME PROJECT IN THE LONG TERM?

Clearly, then, once we have the human gene map, the real work begins. What will we do with it? What are the practical applications? What are the ethical, legal, and social implications of these applications? Some of the major projected outcomes are discussed in the following paragraphs.

Improved Health Care

For many of us, the key question is, "How will all of this information translate into improved health?" The main outcome is expected to be the use of genetic technology to diagnose and predict disease, with the hope that early detection will translate into early intervention. Medicine will be personalized to each individual rather than the "average person" approach presently used.

Insight into Basic Human Biology

In addition to the discovery of specific genes, much insight into how genetic information is stored, retrieved, changed, and connected to an organism's function will issue from the Human Genome Project. Insight into how human beings evolved will be an additional outcome as it becomes possible to compare the human sequence with those of other organisms. Genetics will likely redefine our concepts of race and ethnicity once sequencing is complete.

Improved Technologies

Much progress has already been made in the advancement of laboratory technology used in biological research. Automation, robotics, and advances in computer technology have already been realized and will continue to emerge.

WHAT CAN WE EXPECT OVER THE NEXT DECADE?

As mentioned earlier, completion of the sequencing of the human genome is not an end point, but a beginning in terms of the enormous applications of this information; it is likewise only the beginning of the project's ELSI implications. We have already seen the near-term expected applications of diagnostic testing, pharmacogenomics, and genetics-directed, individualized nutrition therapy. The even more challenging task will be to identify what the segments of DNA actually do. For those sequences that code for proteins, we need to understand how these proteins contribute to the function of cells and how their expression is regulated. For those sequences that are seemingly useless to the cell (the so-called *junk DNA* that makes up the vast majority of the genome of most organisms), we need to understand their role as well. This whole process of understanding the function of the DNA structure is called *annotating* the DNA, assigning a role to each component. All of this new capability opens up increasingly complex questions about how we as a society will handle genetic technology so that it works *for* us rather than *against* us. Expect considerable controversy regarding these applications over the next decade, probably accompanied by legal challenges, as society sorts out the best ways to use this powerful new technology.

Numerous Web sites are helpful in keeping up to date on the project's progress. Refer to the "Useful Web Sites" section at the end of this chapter for several informative sites.

Useful Resources

Collins F, Galas D. A new five-year plan for the U.S. Human Genome Project. *Science.* 1993; 262:43–46.

Collins FS, Jegalian KG. Deciphering the code of life. *Sci Am.* 1999; 281: 86–91.

Collins FS, McKusick VA. Implications of the Human Genome project for medical science. *JAMA.* 2001; 285:540–544.

Collins FS, Patrinos A, Jordan E, Chakravarti A, Gesteland R, Walters L, and the members of the DOE and NIH planning groups. New goals for the U.S. Human Genome Project: 1998-2003. *Science.* 1998; 282:682–689.

Human genomics/genetics. *JAMA.* 2001; 286 (theme issue):2195–2354.

International Human Genome Sequencing Consortium. Initial sequencing and analysis of the human genome. *Nature.* 2001; 409:860–921.

Stephens JC, Schneider JA, Tanguay DA, et al. Haplotype variation and linkage disequilibrium in 313 human genes. *Science.* 2001; 293:489–493.

Strausberg RL, Feingold EA, Klausner RD, Collins FS. The mammalian gene collection. *Science.* 1999; 286:455–457.

Strohman RC. Genomics and human life span—what's left to extend? *Nat Biotechnol.* 2001; 19:195–216.

Venter JC, Adams MD, Myers EW, et al. The sequence of the human genome. *Science.* 2001; 291:1304–1351.

Watson JD, Crick FHC. Molecular structure of nucleic acids: a structure for deoxyribose nucleic acid. *Nature.* 1953; 171:737–738.

Useful Web Sites

Genetics in General

Baker C. Your genes, your choices. Department of Energy Web site. Available at: http://www.ornl.gov/hgmis/publicat/genechoice/index.html. Accessed July 30, 2002.

Casey DK. Genomics and its impact on medicine and society: a 2001 primer. Department of Energy Web site. Available at: http://www.ornl.gov/hgmis/publicat/primer2001/index.html. Accessed July 30, 2002.

Genome watch page. National Center for Biotechnology Information Web site. Available at: http://www.ncbi.nlm.nih.gov/genome/seq. Accessed July 30, 2002.

Hum Genome News [serial online]. Available at: http://www.ornl.gov/hgmis/publicat/hgn/hgn.html. Accessed July 30, 2002.

Modern genetics for all students. Web site of Washington University, St. Louis. Available at: http://www.so.wustl.edu/science_outreach/curriculum/genetics/index.html. Accessed July 30, 2002.

Human Genome Project Gateway Sites

About the Human Genome Project. Department of Energy Web site. Available at: http://www.ornl.gov/hgmis/project/about.html. Accessed July 30, 2002.

Human Genome Project information: ethical, legal, and social issues. Department of Energy Web site. Available at: http://www.ornl.gov/hgmis/elsi/elsi.html. Accessed July 30, 2002.

Human Genome Project information: frequently asked questions. Department of Energy Web site. Available at: http://www.ornl.gov/hgmis/faq/faqs1.html. Accessed July 30, 2002.

Human Genome Project information: topical and alphabetical Web site indexes. Department of Energy Web site. Available at: http://www.ornl.gov/hgmis/toc_expand.html. Accessed July 30, 2002.

Medicine and the new genetics. Department of Energy Web site. Available at: http://www.ornl.gov/hgmis/medicine/medicine.html. Accessed July 30, 2002.

National Human Genome Research Institute page. National Institutes of Health Web site. Available at: http://www.nhgri.nih.gov. Accessed July 30, 2002.

3

Genetic Principles

We have long known that like begets like, that biological information is passed from parent to offspring. This process is called *heredity,* and as we have seen in the previous chapters, the scientific discipline dedicated to studying this complex process is called genetics. Genetics is concerned with how traits are passed from one generation to another, down to the smallest detail of all the processes that must take place in order for traits to be expressed in a particular environment. Genetics as a scientific discipline is evolving into the broader context of genomics as our vision of the important role of genes in the function of the organism within its environment expands. With the growing complexity of this field, it is easy to get mired down in the intricate details and to be unable to separate the key principles from all the detail. This complexity makes genetics appear intimidating, but in fact this science has a set of logical rules followed by all living organisms. In this chapter we will focus on these rules, along with important applications they make possible.

THE RULES: THE MENDELIAN VIEW

No discussion of genetics would be complete without paying tribute to the Austrian monk Gregor Mendel who, as mentioned earlier, is credited with the discovery of the laws of chromosomal inheritance. In the mid-nineteenth century, Mendel experimented with breeding the common garden pea. He created hybrids by crossing plants with dissimilar physical characteristics: tall plants and short plants, plants with green peas and plants with yellow peas, and plants with round peas and plants with wrinkled peas. Plant breeding had been going on for some time before Mendel began his experiments, and it was already known that when plants with dissimilar characteristics were crossed, all the offspring looked alike.

When these offspring were crossed, however, they did not breed true. Instead of producing offspring that all looked like the parents, a mixture of traits was observed—some plants looked like the parents and some like the grandparents. Mendel's genius was in recognizing that there was a pattern to this appearance and disappearance of traits, that a trait was never really lost—it was just hidden. He formalized the rules of passing traits down from generation to generation, and he put forth the concept of trait dominance and recessiveness. When a tall plant is crossed with a short plant, and the progeny is tall, the tall trait is said to be dominant; the trait that is hidden (shortness) is recessive.

How Traits Are Inherited

We now know that Mendel's traits are determined by *genes*, distinct sets of genetic information that are passed from parent to offspring through generation after generation. His rules of inheritance are predictable because genes are located on chromosomes, and chromosomes have set rules for their distribution into the sperm and egg cells that ultimately combine to form the new organism. In the early twentieth century, scientists began to isolate chromosomes and to study what they were made of, how genes were carried on them, and the details of how they were inherited from one generation to the next. This period, known as the era of Mendelian genetics, resulted in important insight into how cells reproduced themselves and their genetic material, as well as how genes were inherited.

Cells as Life's Building Blocks

One of the fundamental concepts of biology is that the cell is the basic unit of life. No matter how small or large the organism, its building blocks are its cells. The simplest forms of life, bacteria, typically have a single cell. More complex organisms, such as trees and human beings, have billions of cells. In such higher organisms, almost all cells have a nucleus, in which the genetic material is housed. If it were arranged end to end, the complete set of genetic information needed to make a human is estimated to be six feet long. In order to package all of that material into the tiny nucleus, however, the genetic material is divided into segments called *chromosomes*. The information for a particular trait is located in a gene somewhere along one of these chromosomes, and in fact, chromosomes are essentially strings of genes arranged one after the other.

The word *chromosome* means "colored body," but chromosomes themselves are virtually colorless. The name comes from the fact that they can be stained in the laboratory, a useful trick for making them visible and for separating them from each other based on their physical size and staining characteristics, a process called *karyotyping*.

Human beings have 23 distinct types of chromosomes. Each has a partner, one member of the pair coming from the mother and one from the father. Of the 23 pairs, 1 pair, composed of the *sex chromosomes*, contains the genes that determine the child's sex: an X and a Y chromosome for a male, two X chromosomes for a female. The other 22 pairs are called *autosomes* and are numbered 1 through 22, with the longest chromosome numbered 1 and the smallest 22. During growth and repair, new cells are formed, and during reproduction, new organisms are formed. In each case there is a precise but different mechanism for ensuring the genetic material is distributed appropriately so that traits can be passed to the new generation.

Mitosis and Meiosis

To create new cells, both partners of each of the chromosomes must be passed from the original cell to the new cell, called the *daughter cell*. This division process is called *mitosis*. Both partners of a chromosome pair are duplicated and distributed to the new cell so that each has a copy of all 46 chromosomes. To create new organisms, however, a special division process called *meiosis* ensures that the genetic material is not doubled when the egg and sperm combine. Only one partner of each chromosome pair goes into the *gamete* (egg or sperm cell in human beings) so that, when the gametes fuse to form the *zygote* (which develops into the fetus), the correct number of chromosomes is restored, and both partners for each chromosome are present. In human beings, then, gametes contain 23 chromosomes, one member of each of the 23 pairs, and the zygote contains the full 46 chromosomes, with a pair of chromosomes for each of the 23.

Phenotypes, Genotypes, Linkage, and Markers

Each partner of a chromosome pair came from a different parent: one member of the pair came from the mother and one from the father. During meiosis, only one member of each chromosome pair will be distributed to the egg or sperm cell. Whether that chromosome originally came from the mother or from the father is usually randomly determined and results in considerable gene shuffling, which explains why children of the same parents are unique, why their *phenotype*–their appearance–is distinct from the parents and from each other: their underlying genes, their *genotypes*, are different. Furthermore, meiosis has a special feature where both chromosomal partners physically pair and can exchange portions of their genetic material, which further increases genetic diversity. Genes that are physically located near each other tend to stay together during this genetic shuffling, and they are said to be linked. A set of *linked genes* is a useful tool in genetic research because the researcher may not know which gene causes the trait of interest but may know that the trait tends to be present whenever another trait appears. The easily detectable trait is called a *marker gene*, or simply a *marker*, and may have nothing to do with the trait of interest. A marker could be another gene responsible for a totally different trait or, more likely, for a short, recognizable sequence of bases. For example, in the early genetic tests for a number of diseases, the disease gene itself was not detected because it was as yet unidentified. What was detected instead was a DNA base change that was present each time that disease was observed. In time, after the gene for the disease was identified and highly specific tests were developed, the original marker was found to be not within the gene itself but so physically close that everywhere the disease gene went, the marker also went. A marker is therefore simply a convenient way of tracking the presence of a gene physically located near the marker but essentially hidden because there is not yet a test that can detect it. When moving genes from one genome to another, molecular biologists prefer markers with easily detectable characteristics, such as resistance to antibiotics.

Genetic Mapping

Linked genes are also essential for developing chromosomal maps. Just as it is possible to physically locate a town on a map of the United States, it is possible to physically locate a gene on a particular chromosome and, further, at a specific position on that chromosome. Mapping involves locating a trait on a specific chromosome, finding a second gene on the same chromosome, and determining the distance between the two genes. By performing the appropriate matings, it is possible to discover how often the two genes stay together. This determination is based on the fact that during reproduction and the formation of the egg and sperm cells, the members of each chromosomal pair physically align along their length and exchange genetic information (discussed above in reference to meiosis). The closer the two linked genes are to each other on the chromosome, the greater the chance that they will stay together and that a genetic exchange will not occur within the distance that separates them. When the offspring of matings in which one parent has both traits and the other has neither are examined, a count is taken of how many offspring contain either both traits or neither trait, which indicates that no genetic exchange has occurred between them, and how many contain either one or the other trait, which means an exchange has occurred. The greater the physical distance between the two traits, the greater the chance an exchange will occur between them and the greater the number of off-spring that will have only a single trait. The shorter the distance, the greater the number of offspring that will have either both traits or neither trait. From this information, the actual distance between the two genes can be calculated.

Obviously this process is tedious, and it takes a lot of time to perform the matings, grow the progeny, analyze their traits, and calculate the distances. Not surprisingly, until the advent of recent technology, progress was slow. When the trait was a human disease, it took quite a while to figure out which trait was responsible and where it was located, a process that gave rise to an understanding of how the trait was inherited and to the ability to predict the chances that an offspring would inherit the disease gene.

Mendelian Inheritance Patterns: Autosomal versus Sex-linked; Dominance versus Recessiveness

In human beings, traits are typically inherited in one of six ways, depending on whether the trait's gene is on an autosome, a sex chromosome, or on the mitochondrial genetic material, and whether the trait is dominant or recessive. Dominance and recessiveness refer to whether a trait is expressed or not. In Mendel's experiments involving the height of the pea plant, for example, crossing a tall plant with a short plant produced all tall plants even though the plants contained both the gene for tall and the gene for short. Tall stature is therefore considered to be displayed, or *dominant*, and short stature is considered to be hidden, or *recessive*, in the presence of tall. Dominance and recessiveness make sense only when a single trait occurs in at least two variations, called *alleles*. If all the plants Mendel had crossed had been tall, tall would always be expressed, making the question of dominance irrelevant, and it would actually be impossible to study the inheritance of tall stature. Thus alleles (variations of a gene) are important tools in genetic research, and they provide the nearly infinite variety observed in the biological world.

The six inheritance patterns are listed below. In the explanations given, the two alleles are the normal and mutant alleles of a gene, and what is being measured is whether the mutant version of a trait is expressed (dominant) or not (recessive):

- Autosomal dominant. Autosomal dominant means the mutant gene is on one of the 22 non-sex-determining chromosome pairs (the autosomes) and that the mutant trait is observable even though the second copy of the gene (its allele) may be normal.
- Autosomal recessive. Autosomal recessive means the mutant gene is on one of the 22 autosomes and that the mutant trait is *not* observed when the normal allele is also present. Only when both alleles are mutant alleles will the mutant trait be observable. For an autosomal recessive trait to be expressed, two mutant copies of the gene must be present.
- X-linked dominant. X-linked means the gene is on the X chromosome. Whether a trait on the X chromosome is dominant or recessive is determined by its expression in women, who have two X chromosomes. Traits on the X chromosome are automatically expressed in men, since only a single copy is present and no measure of dominance or recessiveness can be made. To determine dominance or recessiveness of a trait, women must be carriers, that is, they must have one normal allele and one mutant allele. If the mutant trait is observed, the mutant form of the gene is dominant over the normal version.
- X-linked recessive. In the above example for X-linked dominant, if the mutant allele in carrier females is *not* expressed, then this allele is recessive.
- Y-linked. Males have a single Y chromosome as well as a single X chromosome. As in the situation with the single X, any genes on the Y chromosome will be expressed; the question of dominance is not an issue.
- Mitochondrial. As with the X and Y chromosomes, only a single copy of the mitochondrial DNA exists; dominance and recessiveness do not apply. Mitochondrial inheritance is discussed later in the section titled "Maternal Inheritance."

Homozygotes and heterozygotes   When these inheritance patterns are applied to human disease, they refer to the type of chromosome the disease trait is carried on, either the sex chromosomes or the autosomes, and whether or not the disease is dominant or recessive in the presence of the normal allele.

In autosomal dominant disorders, only one copy of a disease-causing gene needs to be present for the disease to be expressed. With the exception of genes on the X and Y chromosomes in males, where there is only a single copy of each of these chromosomes, each human gene is present in the genome twice, one gene on each of the pair of chromosomes. The gene may occur in its normal form or, if there has been a change in one or more DNA bases, in a mutant form. An individual with either two normal or two mutant alleles at that locus is called a *homozygote*, and the individual is said to be homozygous at that locus. As mentioned earlier, if the individual has one normal and one mutant allele at that locus, the individual is a carrier, a *heterozygote*, and it is said to be heterozygous at that locus.

Penetrance and expressivity   Biology is seldom clear-cut, however. Clear detection of the disease phenotype can be difficult even when an individual carries two genes for the disorder, because the disease state may not be expressed fully. One would expect 100 percent *penetrance*; that is, when someone has two copies of the disease allele, one would expect the disease to be expressed 100 percent of the time. Full penetrance is not always observed, however, for reasons we do not yet understand. A related concept is *expressivity*. If different members of a family all have the mutant gene, but their expression of that gene takes different forms, perhaps varying from mild to severe disease, the gene is said to exhibit variable expressivity. What we are likely seeing here but do not fully understand is the impact of the interaction between environmental factors and gene expression. Even identical twins, having the same DNA, will have variable penetrance and expressivity due to differing interactions with the environments in which they function.

It is this author's suspicion that many of these terms, which have served us well for over a century, were appropriate for the old genetics, when traits were observable and readily described. As we begin to understand the molecular basis for trait inheritance, however, these terms no longer suffice. Dominance and recessiveness will likely be seen as a simplistic way to describe gross morphology and will give way to descriptions of alleles' expressions and their effects, singly and collectively, on that gene's function. The inconsistency with penetrance and expressivity is likely due to the influence of environmental factors on gene expression such that quite different outcomes from the same genes can be possible if those genes are exposed to different communication signals.

Inheritance: Beyond Mendel

Since Mendel's initial discoveries of how single genes were inherited, other inheritance patterns have been observed: the inheritance of the genes on cellular organelles such as the mitochondria (see "Maternal Inheritance" later); differential expression of genes that depend upon which parent contributed the chromosome; and the complex situation involving the inheritance of multiple genes and the influence of multiple factors on the expression of a trait.

Maternal inheritance   In addition to the main set of genetic information in the nucleus, higher organisms such as animals and plants have mitochondria and chloroplasts, organelles that are responsible for cellular energy production and that have their own sets of genetic information. There are also rules for inheriting these sets of information, but they differ from those that govern chromosomes in the nucleus. Specifically, this organellar genetic information is transmitted solely from the female to the offspring, a process called *maternal inheritance.* Human beings have a single copy of circular DNA in the mitochondria believed to have originated from a bacterial infection early in the evolution of higher organisms. All children inherit their mitochondrial DNA from their mothers, a fact that has been useful in tracing the lineage of human beings.

The genes carried on the mitochondrial DNA relate primarily to the organelle's role in oxidative phosphorylation and to the transfer and ribosomal RNA needed for its own housekeeping activities. Interestingly, mutations in mitochondrial DNA can result in the phenotype of diabetes mellitus. How a mitochondrial mutation specifically leads to diabetes is not fully known, but dysfunction in oxidative phosphorylation is suspected of resulting in increased free radical formation that in turn leads to pathogenesis.

Genomic imprinting   According to Mendel's laws of chromosomal inheritance, whether an autosome carrying a defective gene is inherited from the mother or from the father is not important to the expression of a given trait. This seemingly ironclad law of genetics has been shown not to be true in all instances. Recently it has been discovered that two different syndromes result from differences in the expression of the same genetic material on chromosome 15. When the chromosome is inherited from the father, the syndrome manifests as short stature, small hands and feet, poor muscle tone, obesity, mild to moderate mental retardation, and hypogonadism and is called *Prader-Willi syndrome.* When the chromosome is inherited from the mother, the condition is called *Angelman syndrome,* and the symptoms are quite different from Prader-Willi: severe mental retardation, seizures, and ataxia. The basis for the phenotypic difference is the fact that, in the chromosome inherited from the father, certain genes in a specific region of chromosome 15 are expressed (that is, the genetic information is converted from DNA into protein), whereas in the chromosome inherited from the mother, these same genes are not expressed. Conversely, certain other genes in this region are expressed in the chromosome inherited from the mother but not in the chromosome inherited from the father. The net result is that, for several genes, only one of the two copies in a given individual is expressed. If that copy of the gene is lost through a deletion of the critical region of chromosome 15 or through improper gamete formation such that no copies of the chromosome end up in the sperm or egg cell, the genetic information from that gene is lost, preventing its normal protein production, and disease results. This phenomenon of differential expression depending on which parent supplies the gene is called *genomic imprinting*. Molecular techniques such as those detailed in Chapter 4 have made it possible to identify genes and their products and to understand how the loss of these products results in the different phenotypes observed.

Multigenic and multifactorial inheritance   Clearly, gene expression is a complex process that varies with the particular gene and the environment in which it is expressed. Fully understanding diseases caused by changes in a single gene, a straightforward process compared with understanding today's chronic diseases, is an ongoing challenge in itself. These chronic diseases, such as atherosclerosis, obesity, diabetes, and cancer, are even more challenging because there are a number of genes involved (multigenic) and because their expression is strongly influenced by a number of lifestyle factors (multifactorial). At this early stage of understanding, scientists must talk about genetic susceptibility and modifiable risk factors in lieu of identifying which genes are involved, what they do, and how environmental factors such as nutrition can influence their impact on health. Unraveling the complexity of chronic disease genes and the factors that influence their expression is a major goal of the Human Genome Project, however, and the next decade should yield considerable information.

THE RULES: THE MOLECULAR VIEW

The first part of the twentieth century saw significant progress in the development of the science of genetics and in understanding how chromosomes and the traits (genes) they carried were inherited. In the 1950s

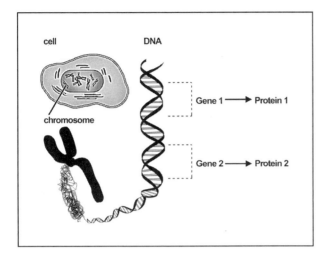

Figure 3-1
Interrelationship among chromosomes, DNA, genes, and proteins.

Chromosomes in the nucleus of cells contain the genetic material DNA (deoxyribonucleic acid), which in turn contains genes, DNA sequences that are translated into proteins that serve as enzymes, hormones, receptors, communication molecules, and such.

the focus began to shift to understanding the composition of genes and chromosomes, how information was stored and retrieved, and the details of genes specifically associated with diseases.

For many years scientists thought protein was the genetic material. Gradually, however, experiments pointed conclusively toward DNA. In 1953 James Watson and Francis Crick, using the x-ray crystallography data of Rosalind Franklin and Maurice Wilkins, deduced the structure of this substance. This work showed how the unique properties of DNA could explain the inheritance characteristics of chromosomes, which led scientists to accept that DNA, not protein, was the genetic material. Through their work we have come to understand the relationship among chromosomes, DNA bases, and cellular proteins (Figure 3-1).

DNA as a Source of Encoded Information That Must Be Stored and Retrieved

DNA contains information that directs the synthesis of all the life-sustaining activities of the organism. The DNA molecule is made up of four chemical compounds called nucleotides, which consist of the nitrogenous bases adenine (A), guanine (G), cytosine (C), and thymine (T), plus phosphate and the sugar deoxyribose. The structures of the bases allow for weak hydrogen bonding between specific pairs – A pairs with T and G with C – to form a double helix. To better understand the shape of this molecule, picture a spiral staircase, with the sugar-phosphate backbone of the DNA forming the parallel railings and the paired bases forming the steps that connect them.

DNA is encoded information that tells a story. As the text is read, an organized, logical description unfolds as to how to make the myriad of proteins needed to build the organism and support its functions. Like any code or language, there is an underlying organization: a set of symbols or letters that are assembled into words, sentences, chapters, books, and ultimately a complete encyclopedia of information (Table 3-1). The bases A, G, C, and T are the letters of this code. These bases are arranged side by side to form a linear molecule. Words are created by "reading" three bases at a time, a unit called a *codon*. Sets of three bases ultimately direct the positioning of a particular amino acid into the protein molecule being assembled. Each codon specifies one of the 20 or so amino acids that make up the various proteins. Changes in the spelling of a word can result in a change in the directions for inserting the correct amino acid into the protein being assembled. Such genetic misspellings are called *mutations.*

A gene is the set of sequential codons required to synthesize a protein, and it is analogous to a sentence. Like a sentence, a gene has a characteristic syntax. Instead of a subject, verb, and predicate, genes have start (initiation), coding (informational), and stop (termination) sequences. DNA has many genes arranged along its length. Just as the total sentence content in a book is divided into chapters, DNA is subdivided into units called chromosomes. And, just as a book is the sum total of all its chapters, the genome is the sum total of all the genetic material, that which is known to be informational, and the remainder, which is currently considered to be noninformational.

A fundamental principle of genetics is that each cell's nucleus contains the complete genome for the organism, even though the information may

Table 3-1 The Language of DNA	
English Language Term	**Genetic Counterpart**
Letter	A[denine], T[hymine], C[ytosine], G[uanine]
Word	Codon
Sentence	Gene
Chapter	Chromosome
Book	Genome

not all be used by a particular cell type. Liver cells use different subsections of genetic information than do heart cells or brain cells. Think of the genome as an encyclopedia. To learn about a topic we do not need to read the whole encyclopedia; we just need to go to a section and retrieve that specific information. Similarly, to carry out a particular function, a cell needs to read (translate) only certain sections of the total book (the genome).

Another fundamental principle is that the language of DNA is common to all organisms, whether microbes, plants, or animals. Species differ in their individual encyclopedias. The content is different, but the code and methods of decoding are the same for all; that is why scientists can study the fruit fly or roundworm and uncover fundamental principles that also apply to human beings.

If the genetic material of all organisms is basically the same, and members of a species share an even greater percentage of identical DNA sequences, why don't we all look alike? Returning to the book analogy, it is helpful to think of individual differences as resulting from individual authors attempting to write the same chapter for the encyclopedia. If we give ten authors the same outline for a chapter, they will write the sentences for that chapter slightly differently to express the same basic concepts. The meaning of many concepts will still be clear in spite of slight variations. Other concepts will be lost altogether. Similarly, many genes can accommodate one or more misspellings that result in slight variations, yet still produce a functional protein; this protein may be as functional as, less functional than, or even more functional than the original version. Other genes cannot accommodate even a single misspelling. In molecular terms, these misspellings are mutations that are the cornerstone of evolution. Genes that cannot accommodate change are said to be highly conserved and usually code for proteins that are critical to the functioning of the organism. Other genes can more readily accommodate change and often exist in a number of subtle variations ultimately responsible for the differences among individuals within a species. Every member of the species uses the same basic blueprint; they simply go about building and maintaining their houses slightly differently so that the end results reflect their individual characters.

The Molecular Biology of DNA

Molecular biology is the study of the decoding of DNA, how the sequence of bases is converted into protein components such as enzymes, hormones, messenger molecules, receptors, and so on that are useful to the cell. Transferring the information in the DNA sequence into a protein requires two major steps: transcription and translation. The DNA sequence is transcribed into an RNA sequence, which is in turn translated into an amino acid sequence. In the nucleus, the DNA double helix unzips itself, and RNA polymerase enzymes move along a strand, matching bases in complementary pairing fashion to the linear sequence of bases in the DNA. The RNA molecule that is formed is called messenger RNA (mRNA). RNA is similar to DNA except that it does not contain thymine (T); instead it uses the base uracil (U) to pair with adenine (A).

Genes have a standard anatomy (Figure 3-2). Upstream from the informational region is a regulatory region where RNA polymerase binds (the *promoter region*) and where a variety of factors, including environmental factors such as nutrients, can bind directly or indirectly to turn on or off the expression of that gene. Then comes the informational region (known as the *coding region* or *structural gene*), followed by a stop region. Similar to reading an encyclopedia, RNA polymerase does not read the entire DNA just to make a particular protein; it transcribes only the genes needed by the cell at a particular time.

Within the coding region of a gene, interspersed in the information sequences, are sequences that are noncoding, that is, those that do not translate into proteins. In molecular biology terminology, DNA sequences containing information that translates into the amino acid sequence of a protein are called *exons*. The intervening sequences are called *introns*. RNA polymerase transcribes the entire gene into mRNA, both the coding and noncoding regions. Predictably, following transcription there is a processing step called posttranscriptional processing. Enzymes remove the introns from the message, a run of adenine bases is attached, and the mRNA is transported from the nucleus to the cytoplasm, where it is translated into protein.

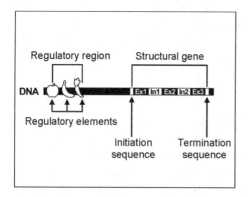

Figure 3-2   Anatomy of a gene.

Abbreviations: DNA, deoxyribonucleic acid; Ex, exon; In, intron.

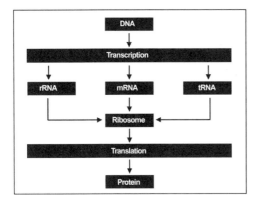

Figure 3-3   Flow of information from DNA to protein.

Abbreviations: mRNA, messenger ribonucleic acid; rRNA, ribosomal ribonucleic acid; tRNA, transfer ribonucleic acid.

In the cytoplasm, the mRNA attaches to ribosomal RNA (rRNA), and one codon at a time systematically directs the assembly of amino acid molecules into a protein. The protein may be ready to go at this point, or before it is an active molecule it may require posttranslational processing such as adding sugars or cleaving it into a smaller molecule. Familiar examples include the posttranslational cleaving of proenzymes such as pepsinogen, trypsinogen, and insulin, as well as the addition of a carbohydrate functional group to glycoproteins. The finished protein then spontaneously assumes the structural shape needed for the molecule to function. Figure 3-3 provides an overview of the decoding of the genetic information into protein.

The information represented by the base sequence of DNA is translated into a protein product. Thus mutations in the DNA will ultimately be converted into changes in proteins. Changes in the coding region are more likely to have harmful effects on function and lead to a disease state than changes in the introns, those presumably noninformational sequences within the gene, or in the intervening sequences that separate a gene from its neighbor.

Genotype versus Phenotype and Dominance versus Recessiveness, at the Molecular Level

A gene is found at a specific location on a chromosome called a *locus* (plural *loci*). There are two alleles of each gene, one on each member of the chromosome pair and located at the same position on the two chromosomes. The information in the two copies is the genotype for that particular gene; the end product that results from the expression of that information and the measurable impact it has on the cell is the phenotype for that gene.

The genotype and phenotype can be compared to a music CD. Usually the music encoded in the CD is translated and expressed from the first track through to the last. Outside influences, such as programming the CD player to select tracks at random or repeatedly playing just one track, change the outcomes that flow from the CD. The music embedded in the CD has not changed, however—only its expression has changed. Similarly, the genetic information simply encodes information, the genotype. How that information is expressed, which can be influenced by a number of factors, determines the phenotype.

Only phenotypes can be dominant or recessive. Genes themselves are not dominant or recessive; the effects they produce are. The concepts of dominance and recessiveness are straightforward when one talks about physical traits: one copy's effects dominate the other in an all-or-none fashion. Brown eye color is considered a dominant trait in brown-eyed parents with a blue-eyed child. Blue eye color is recessive. The brown-eyed parents are carriers, having one allele for the gene coding for brown eye color and one for blue eye color. The phenotype is brown eye color, but the genotype is brown/blue. The parents are heterozygous for eye color. Since brown is dominant to blue (or, from the opposite perspective, blue is recessive to brown), the child must have two alleles that code for blue eye color (that is, he or she must be homozygous for blue eye color) in order to have blue eyes.

According to this earlier thinking, an abnormality (such as a disease) was thought to result only when both copies of the gene were mutated and function was severely impaired. The heterozygous individual, with one normal and one abnormal allele each, was considered to be functionally normal. Genetic disease was therefore considered rare. As long as one normal copy of that gene was present, some active protein was produced, severe dysfunction was prevented, and the disease, as it had been defined, was not evident. As our level of technological sophistication has increased, and we have learned what the gene product is and how to detect it, it has become obvious that in the carrier individual, one normal gene product and one mutant gene product are present; such individuals can have a functional level less than normal but not severely dysfunctional. Increasing focus is now being directed to detecting the carrier individual and assessing whether having one normal and one mutant gene impairs function and increases the risk of developing disease. What is expected to emerge is a gradation of functions, depending on the nature of the mutation and the specific effect on the protein's function. The majority of people are likely heterozygous at any given gene locus, which suggests that most clients we see may be heterozygous and have less than normal (that is, some degree of impaired) function.

THE RULES: THE GENOMIC VIEW

With the advent of the Human Genome Project, genetics is rapidly evolving into the broader vision known as genomics, a more global approach than studying just the inheritance of traits or the molecular basis for such inheritance. Genetics in this context will focus on even more complex issues, while at the same time addressing fundamental ones: how many genes we (and other organisms) have, what these genes do, how cells work, how a single cell develops into a complex organism, how single genes cause disease, how multiple genes interact to cause disease, how to develop diagnostic tests to provide early means of detection and intervention, and how communication takes place between genetic material and the environment. Broader questions include how human genetic makeup compares with that of other organisms, how living things have evolved, how closely related various species are, and whether the concepts of speciation and race make sense when considered at the genetic level.

For the most part, we do not know what the rules will be. We do know that having the details of the entire genome available will cause fundamental changes in what scientists and clinicians will be able to do. For clinicians, the genomic view will be one of a personalized and gene-directed approach for keeping each individual well.

Useful Resources

Horowitz M. *Basic Concepts in Medical Genetics*. New York, NY: McGraw-Hill Book Co; 2000.

Jorde LB, Carey JC, Bamshad MJ, White RL. *Medical Genetics*. St. Louis, Mo: Mosby Inc; 2000.

Klug WS, Cummings MR. *Concepts of Genetics*. 6th ed. Upper Saddle River, NJ: Prentice Hall Inc; 2000.

Lewin B. *Genes VII*. New York, NY: Oxford University Press; 1999.

Snustad DP, Simmons MJ. *Principles of Genetics*. 2nd ed. New York, NY: John Wiley & Sons Inc; 1999.

Thompson MW, McInnes RR, Huntington FW. *Genetics in Medicine*. 5th ed. Philadelphia, Pa: WB Saunders Co; 1999.

Useful Web Sites

Basic genetics/genomics. National Institutes of Health, Division of Intramural Research's Office of Science Education and Outreach Web site. Available at: http://www.nhgri.nih.gov/DIR/VIP. Accessed July 31, 2002.

Genetics and Genomics on the Web. National Institutes of Health Web site. Available at: http://www.nhgri.nih.gov/Data. Accessed July 31, 2002.

Genomics and Its Impact on Medicine and Society: A 2001 Primer. Available at: http://www.ornl.gov/hgmis/publicat/primer2001. Accessed July 31, 2002.

Office of Genetics and Disease Prevention page. Centers for Disease Control and Prevention Web site. Available at: http://www.cdc.gov/genetics/. Accessed July 31, 2002.

4

Genetic Technologies

T he Human Genome Project is a highly technical effort that relies on a variety of genctic technologies. Many technologies that worked well in the laboratory were available when the project began, but they needed further development to increase their accuracy and efficiency and to reduce their cost before they were useful for such a large-scale effort. Additionally, new technologies and new technological fields were needed.

Excellent, steady progress has been made in improving existing technologies and developing new ones, to the extent that they significantly expanded the vision of the types of problems that genetic research could tackle and greatly expanded the scope of the Human Genome Project itself. Many more new and improved technologies are expected to continue to be forthcoming as research progresses.

It is important for those working in fields affected by developments in genetic research to understand the fundamental technologies used. The rapid pace of technology development and the complexity of today's genetic research make understanding the intricacies of the various technologies a daunting task. Fortunately, the underlying goals of genetic research are not too different from those that have been at the forefront since Mendel's time. It is the methods, rather than the fundamentals, that have changed and become more sophisticated. By constructing a clear framework of what genetic research is trying to accomplish, regardless of the intricacies of the technologies and specific techniques used, it is easy to grasp the fundamental concepts and terminology, which will provide a basis from which to build understanding of new technologies as they develop.

The fundamental goals of genetic research include the following:

- **To visualize the genetic material.** What does it look like; how is it organized; is the right amount present and in the proper orientation?

- **To define the basic steps involved in storing and retrieving genetic information.** What is the nature of the molecule that stores the genetic information; how is the information encoded in that molecule; how is it extracted from that molecule and converted into something useful at the cellular level; how is this information transmitted to new generations; and how does the genetic makeup of one organism differ from another?
- **To map genes to particular locations on chromosomes.** Where does a particular gene reside; how is it transmitted to subsequent generations; and how can this information be used to predict risk to individuals within a family?
- **To identify the product of each gene and its function.** What does each gene translate into; how does the gene product contribute to the health of the organism; what types of errors can occur; and what happens when errors are made, and dysfunction results?
- **To understand how the expression of each gene's information is controlled.** How is each gene's expression turned on and off mechanically; what are the signals that communicate with the genes and influence expression; and what options do we have for altering expression therapeutically?
- **To apply the fundamental genetic principles that emerge from research.** What are the best ways to translate these principles into practical applications that will improve the quality of life for citizens worldwide?
- **To improve food crop production.** How can plant and animal breeding be improved so that the quantity and quality of food production are enhanced?
- **To improve health care for human beings and animals.** How can basic research be converted into tools that can be used to predict and to detect disease early as well as to ameliorate and to potentially cure it?

This chapter will focus on developing a working knowledge of technologies central to genetic research. Technologies that have been key to the progress of a particular goal of genetic research or that are commonly encountered in food- and nutrition-related genetic research have been selected for emphasis here. The area of biology that applies genetic technologies to living organisms is called *biotechnology*. Biotechnology is often perceived as separate from genetics, but it's not. This field is concerned with the practical applications of biological organisms or their subcellular components, such as enzymes. Until recently, the field has been limited primarily to water and waste treatment processes and to fermentation processes such as the making of beer, bread, and cheese using enzymes produced by microorganisms. With the development of recombinant DNA technology and monoclonal antibody technology, however, biotechnology has been able to expand its reach into a broader range of food production, health-related, and environmental applications. The key technologies responsible for this expansion of biotechnology and its present-day applications are discussed throughout this chapter.

VISUALIZING THE GENETIC MATERIAL

Imagine how perplexing it must have been to suspect that there was a tangible entity that could be passed from generation to generation, which was ultimately responsible for a disease, but not to be able to see that entity. We now realize that these tangible entities are genes carried on chromosomes. The ability to isolate and stain chromosomes so that they become visible under a microscope was a significant step forward in genetic research. The process involves isolating nucleated cells from an individual and growing them in the laboratory in a culture medium. After many cell divisions have produced a large number of cells, an inhibiting agent is added to the culture to halt the cells at certain stages of division at which the chromosomes are condensed enough to be visible under a microscope when stained.

Karyotyping

Valuable applications of the ability to make chromosomes visible include counting the chromosomes from each cell to ensure that the full number is present, taking a picture of the chromosomes from single cells, and assembling the chromosomes manually (or, more recently, by computer) into a karyotype, in which the chromosomes are paired and arranged in order of size from longest to shortest, with the X and Y chromosomes at the end. Karyotypes are useful for determining whether each chromosome is present in the correct number of copies and whether the gross structure of each chromosome is characteristic of that chromosome (i.e., "normal"). When dyes are used that can stain certain regions of each chromosome but not others, a banded appearance is generated and, from this pattern, it is possible to determine that the fine structure of each chromosome corresponds to the normal arrangement of the genetic material from one end of the chromosome to the other. Maintaining this arrangement unchanged is important because the correct translation of the information in the genes along a chromosome depends on a specific side-by-side arrangement of the DNA bases.

Fluorescence in Situ Hybridization

Fluorescence in situ hybridization (FISH) is an improvement on these early visualization techniques and is commonly used to detect deletions or additions of genetic material within a chromosome or translocation of a part of one chromosome onto another. The FISH technique makes use of DNA probes, which will be discussed in more detail later in this chapter. A fragment of DNA that can recognize a specific region of a particular chromosome is synthesized and has a fluorescent dye incorporated into it. When that DNA fragment (called a *probe*) finds the particular chromosomal region that it recognizes, it binds to that region and can be detected by fluorescence that is now attached to that chromosome.

Spectral Karyotyping

Spectral karyotyping is a further enhancement of the FISH technique. For each chromosome, multiple DNA probes are used that can bind to different regions of a particular chromosome. Multiple colors of fluorescent dyes are used to tag these probes, one color per chromosome, so that each chromosome is a different color. Using this technique, all forty-six chromosomes can be seen at one time. Spectral karyotyping is particularly useful for detecting changes in the normal structure of chromosomes not detectable by traditional methods. For example, breaks in the DNA within a chromosome are possible. A single break could result in a piece of one chromosome breaking away and attaching to the end of another chromosome, which is called a *translocation.* Two breaks in the DNA may cause a segment of the chromosome to be lost, or that segment may reinsert itself into the chromosome but in a different orientation (a process called *rearrangement*). Since chromosomes are made up of a continuous DNA molecule subdivided into thousands of genes, the rearrangement of the genetic information usually has profound effects on the organism's ability to function. Spectral karyotyping can pick up many of these types of changes.

Practical applications of karyotyping include prenatal diagnosis of various disorders, amniocentesis, chorionic villus sampling (CVS), and cancer diagnostics. Amniocentesis and CVS both involve withdrawing fetal cells, culturing them in the laboratory, and analyzing the fetal chromosomes to detect abnormalities. Amniocentesis, the original prenatal sampling, is done during the second trimester, whereas CVS, a more recent development, allows analysis during the first trimester. Cancer is characterized by changes in the chromosomal composition of the cells such that the cells of a tumor ultimately have a characteristic chromosomal profile. Karyotyping can help to identify cancer cell types and to stage the cancer. For example, analysis of the number of changes in the chromosomes and the specific nature of the changes can help to predict the severity of the cancer and direct the therapy.

Spectral karyotyping can also pick up subtle differences that would be missed with traditional staining. For example, a couple who have a mildly retarded child and who are considering another pregnancy were concerned that their second child would also be mentally retarded. Mental retardation is commonly seen when there is an extra amount of chromosomal material, which can vary from an extra whole chromosome to just a tiny portion of one. Knowing this, the clinician ordered a karyotype of the child to see whether a chromosomal abnormality was present. Conventional staining showed no problems; spectral karyotyping, however, detected two normal chromosome 11s, which were blue, and a blue speck (indicative of chromosome 11) on the tip of chromosome 1, which was yellow. A tiny portion of chromosome 11 had been translocated to the tip of chromosome 1. Since the child also had two normal chromosome 11s with their full genetic information, the extra segment of chromosome 11 gave him three copies of that portion of the chromosome. Duplication of one or more genes in that segment was presumably responsible for the mild mental retardation. The parents were then tested, and the father was found to have the same translocation; he was not, however, mentally retarded. On close examination, it was apparent that he had two copies of chromosome 11, one normal chromosome 11 and one in which the tip had broken away and attached itself to the tip of chromosome 1. This condition is called a *balanced translocation*, and he was fortunate that having the genetic material relocated in this way apparently did not impair his functioning. The couple was then counseled as to the probability of further offspring inheriting the extra chromosomal material and developing mental retardation.

In addition to the improved detection of chromosomal abnormalities that these new approaches offer, they also allow for automation. A computer can sort the chromosomes by size and color and generate a karyotype faster and more accurately than the typical manual method. Automation will be increasingly necessary as genetic analysis becomes commonplace and the number of diagnostic karyotypes analyzed each year (currently approximately a half million) increases.

DECIPHERING THE MYSTERIES OF INFORMATION STORAGE AND RETRIEVAL

Over the past five decades, genetic research has focused on solving the mysteries of the chemical nature of the genetic material: how it's copied and distributed to each new cell, how information is stored in the sequence of bases that make up DNA, how the information is extracted from the DNA and converted into proteins, and what the functional consequences are to the cell when errors are made in any of these processes. The basics of these processes were discussed in Chapter 3.

Recombinant DNA Technology

From this basic research have come a number of technical advances that have led to the modern era of genomics. Chief among them is *recombinant DNA* (rDNA) *technology*, also called *genetic engineering*. The development of rDNA technology was revolutionary because it greatly expanded what genetic research could do, the precision with which it could be done, and how quickly it could be done. Recombinant DNA technology was developed in the early 1970s, and its applications to biotechnology in terms of basic science, health care, and food production were readily apparent. Three decades later we have many improvements in plant and animal breeding, new approaches to medical diagnostics, therapeutic tools never before possible, and, ultimately, the ability to conceive and successfully execute a project of the magnitude of the Human Genome Project.

Recombinant DNA has enabled the construction of new genetic combinations, a powerful technological breakthrough that has greatly accelerated the pace of genetic research. It has also given rise to many applications that will soon be commonplace in medical therapy and that will be discussed in detail in the next chapter: DNA-based diagnostic testing, drug responder and nonresponder profiling, therapeutic proteins, and the potential for correcting errors in the genetic material of an individual through gene therapy.

The ability to construct new genetic combinations is at the heart of much of present-day genetic technology. The cornerstone discovery that paved the way to rDNA technology was the discovery of bacterial enzymes called *restriction enzymes* (or *restriction endonucleases*). In bacteria, restriction enzymes serve a defense function: they restrict the entry of foreign DNA into the organism. Various different enzymes protect bacteria from viruses and other sources of invading DNA. Each enzyme is specific for a certain DNA base sequence and cuts the DNA at that specific sequence. By cutting the foreign DNA, the enzymes disrupt its encoded message and prevent it from taking over the bacterium's metabolic machinery. In the laboratory, investigators can use these enzymes as molecular scissors and systematically disassemble and reassemble the genetic material, a process that has been important for deciphering the basic organization of DNA. Being able to cut and paste genetic material at will also allows researchers to remove genetic material from one chromosome and place it into another, as well as to select genetic material from one organism and put it into an unrelated organism.

Why was this ability to manipulate the genetic material revolutionary, and how is it useful? Remember that in nature the ability to create new combinations of genetic information is limited by whether or not the two organisms contributing the genetic material can mate sexually. Since bacteria and human beings are not normal bedfellows, the ability to make hybrid genetic material that combined the gene for human insulin with the rapid growth and gene expression capability of bacteria was not even a remote possibility prior to the development of recombinant DNA technology. With rDNA technology, a high degree of control over the genetic manipulation process is possible. The process can be done precisely and in a fraction of the time required by conventional breeding.

Not only can the genetic makeup of an organism be custom engineered (assumedly to some beneficial end—more on this in a moment), but diagnostic tools can also be developed that would not be possible using conventional methods. For example, you may have engineered a bacterium so that it grows exceptionally well in a large-scale industrial setting and produces a high yield of protein. Into this background you want to insert genes that code for various human therapeutic proteins. You want to be able to cut and paste a fragment of DNA that codes for a human therapeutic protein, no more and no less, into that bacterium without disrupting the desirable growth and production characteristics of the bacterium. You would not be able to produce such a therapeutic protein-generating bacterial factory using conventional means and, even if you could, the probability is high that you would trade out part of the genetic material related to growth and productivity in exchange for the new material coming in.

Similarly, you might want to increase the lycopene content of a tomato with gorgeous red color and fantastic flavor. You could conceivably develop such a tomato using conventional breeding methods, but you would have to cross the plants, collect the seeds, plant the seeds, and test a very large number of seedlings before finding a plant that combined all three characteristics in the same tomato. With recombinant DNA technology, it's possible to insert a regulatory element and increase the expression of the genes involved with lycopene synthesis while maintaining the desirable color and flavor already found in that tomato's genetic material.

Recombinant DNA technology has paved the way for the development of several innovative advances in genetic research:

■ Genetically engineered bacteria and other organisms that could be used to make therapeutic proteins, such as enzymes, hormones, and blood clotting factors; to amplify the amount of a DNA sequence such that there is sufficient material to study; and to investigate the regulation of gene expression by cutting and pasting DNA sequences containing information that can be translated into proteins and the sequences that control this translation

■ Gene cloning, which involves cutting and pasting a gene into another organism's genetic material to make new genetic combinations, to generate large quantities of the gene in order to study its properties, and to construct experimental systems whereby the regulation of the expression of a genetic sequence can be investigated

■ Useful genetic tools, such as

— DNA probes, which can be used for gene mapping, risk prediction, disease detection, drug utilization profiling, identification purposes, or the detection of genetic variation among individuals

— DNA amplification, either by cloning or polymerase chain reaction

— DNA sequencing, which can be used for gene mapping and disease detection

— DNA typing for the purposes of identifying individuals by their genetic fingerprints

■ Methods for comparing the genetic similarity and variation among a wide variety of organisms, referred to as *comparative genomics*

■ Mapping genes to their chromosomal locations
■ Identifying gene products and examining their role in the functioning of a given organism
■ Food production and health care–related applications:
— Transgenic technology, in which genes from one species are introduced into another species, providing a rapid and precise approach to developing food plants and animals that address the limitations in current food crops, from nutritional composition to limitations on production output
— Diagnostic tests and genotype profiling used for disease prediction and diagnosis as well as risk assessment
— Diagnostic tests used for food safety applications
— Therapeutic proteins, particularly those that are in limited supply or not available at all
— Gene therapy, in which a segment of DNA containing a mutation in its sequence of bases can be replaced with the normal sequence

The significance and practical application of these various advances follow.

Genetically engineered organisms   Genetically engineered organisms contain a DNA sequence introduced through the cut-and-paste techniques of recombinant DNA technology described earlier. Organisms ranging from viruses to simple microorganisms such as bacteria, yeast, and other fungi to the more complex plants and animals can be genetically engineered using this technology. Typically, the sequence introduced is not native to the host organism and comes from an altogether different species of organism (such as a human gene introduced into a bacterium's or a mouse's genetic material). Such manipulations are called *transgenic*–that is, they introduce genes across species–and we have thus come to have two terms to describe organisms with cut-and-pasted genetic material: genetically engineered organisms and transgenic organisms. Typically, lower organisms are described as genetically engineered (bacteria, viruses, fungi), and higher organisms are described as transgenic (plants and animals). This book will observe this convention, and this section will focus on recombinant DNA technology as it applies to the genetic engineering of lower organisms. See a later section in this chapter, "Genetic tools: transgenic organism technology," for a discussion of genetic engineering in plants and animals.

Organisms such as bacteria, viruses, and fungi are genetically engineered for a number of reasons. In some cases experimental systems can be constructed so that the role of a gene's product in the functioning of an organism or the details of how the gene's expression is controlled can be studied in the laboratory. Alternatively, the genetically engineered organism may simply be used as a vector that carries within its own genetic material a foreign DNA sequence to be amplified or to be transferred to another cell. Common vectors are viruses or special circular DNA molecules called plasmids. Like restriction enzymes, plasmids are normal components of bacteria. They are separate from the main bacterial DNA and often occur in multiple copies. Vectors differ in the amount of DNA they can incorporate; viruses typically can accept larger fragments than plasmids can.

One of the first applications of genetically engineered organisms was to amplify DNA sequences so that researchers had sufficient quantity for experimentation. Each time the organism multiplies, it makes another copy of the foreign DNA that it contains. Another early application was to insert genes that coded for proteins with commercial value, such as clot-busting enzymes, interferons for fighting viral infections, protein hormones such as insulin and growth hormone, and other proteins useful for food production and environmental applications. The genetically engineered organisms became protein-generating factories because every time the organism copied and expressed its DNA, the foreign gene was also copied and expressed.

In addition to their usefulness in increasing the number of copies of a DNA sequence, recombinant DNA vectors can be used to transfer a DNA sequence from one organism to another, a technical feat that is critical to successful gene therapy. A number of technical tools are required: DNA probes to identify the normal gene sequence, restriction enzymes as well as separation and recovery technology to isolate the DNA sequence, amplification to increase the number of copies of the sequence, and a vector to deliver the sequence to cells that can then incorporate it in exchange for the dysfunctional sequence. Viruses are theoretically promising vectors for gene therapy because they can accept large fragments of DNA, and they come equipped with the ability to infect cells and incorporate their own DNA, as well as any foreign DNA they are carrying, into the recipient cell's DNA.

Gene cloning   Cloning is the ability to make multiple identical copies of something: a piece of DNA, a microorganism, a plant, or an animal. Cloning is usually associated with modern biotechnology, but it has actually been practiced for quite some time. Pure cultures of microorganisms and their viruses are maintained by cloning–growing the original organisms under conditions that allow them to divide and produce genetically identical copies of themselves. Each time a cutting from a plant is grown into a new, genetically identical plant, that original plant has been cloned. Today, however, the term *cloning* can also refer to amplifying a DNA sequence to increase the yield of the protein coded for by that sequence. The terms *gene cloning* and *molecular cloning* are sometimes used to distinguish the cloning of DNA sequences from the cloning of plants or animals, such as the recent cloning of animals.

Genetic tools: DNA probes Restriction enzymes have been important to the development of genetic probes. DNA containing a sequence of interest is cut with restriction enzymes, the fragments are isolated and converted into single strands, and they are then used as templates to synthesize complementary DNA strands. One of the bases used during the copying process has radioactivity or fluorescence attached to it so that the newly synthesized DNA strand is tagged and can be tracked. That strand can then be used to probe a set of single-stranded fragments made from the entire human genome and to identify the fragment that contains the gene of interest. The labeled DNA fragment binds, following the rules of complementary base pairing, to the stretch of DNA complementary to its own base sequence. After unbound DNA is washed away, the fragment that binds the labeled DNA probe can be identified and isolated. DNA probe technology provides a major tool for identifying genes and their chromosomal locations, for detecting disease, and for identifying organisms from bacteria to human beings.

Using DNA probes for identification purposes has many applications. In the medical laboratory they can be used to distinguish between closely related organisms or cell types, which affects the therapy chosen. For example, using DNA probes specific to particular infectious microorganisms allows for rapid differentiation and the start of appropriate therapy. Similarly, cancer tumors may look alike morphologically but be quite different in their therapeutic responses. DNA probes can distinguish the various tumor types and direct the therapy appropriately.

DNA probes can also be used to detect the genetic uniqueness between individuals, which forms the basis for distinguishing the identity of one person from another. In forensics, such DNA "fingerprints" are now routinely used to identify the perpetrator of a crime. DNA probes (autosomal microsatellites), along with DNA sequencing and amplification technologies (discussed below), were useful in the recent identification of members of the Russian royal family of Czar Nicholas II and his wife Alexandra. The family had reputedly been murdered, but only recently were bodies recovered from the putative murder site and identified as members of the royal family through modern genetic techniques. The basis for identification and gene profiling technology using DNA probes is discussed in the sections "Genetic tools: DNA typing" and "Comparative Genomics."

Genetic tools: DNA amplification   A single copy of a DNA sequence is much too small an amount of material to be useful from an experimental standpoint; therefore that single copy must be amplified into thousands of copies. It may sound like an easy feat to isolate the entire genome and then make as many copies as needed. The best we can do at this point, however, is to make multiple copies of small fragments. Initially, DNA amplification was carried out using vectors such as the bacteria and viruses previously described in the section "Genetically engineered organisms." This approach is called *in vivo DNA amplification.*

Amplification of most small DNA fragments is now done primarily using laboratory equipment rather than vectors, through the technique of *polymerase chain reaction* (PCR), which can be thought of as amplification in vitro. For example, a genetic test to determine whether someone is at risk for developing a disease uses a set of DNA probes that can detect the common mutations in the gene associated with the disease. Large quantities of these DNA probes are required for these tests, and they are synthesized using PCR. This technique was so critical to the progress of DNA research that it earned its developer, Kary Mullis, Ph.D., the Nobel Prize in chemistry in 1993. Using nature's basic process of duplicating DNA, Mullis developed a molecular photocopying process in which the number of copies of the DNA fragment would double each time the reaction was run: 2 copies, then 4, 8, 16, 32, 64, and so on. His insight led to the present-day automated process whereby over a billion low-cost copies of a segment of DNA can be made in just hours.

Polymerase chain reaction has been a major technological breakthrough for molecular biology research, without which the Human Genome Project would not have been possible, because literally millions of copies of each DNA fragment are required, and the time and cost of producing such a quantity of DNA manually would have been prohibitive. This method of copying DNA also plays a major role in DNA-based identification technologies such as the use of minute amounts of DNA found in fossils or mummies or in a blood or hair sample from a crime scene. PCR can amplify the amount of DNA so that even a tiny DNA fragment is useful for identification purposes (see section titled "Genetics tools: DNA typing").

Genetic tools: DNA sequencing   DNA sequencing involves identifying, in order, the bases that make up a region of DNA. For example, you may have isolated the gene that codes for blood-clotting factor VIII, the protein missing in individuals with hemophilia A, a severe bleeding disorder. You will want to know the gene's sequence because it will provide information about the size of the gene, the control region that comes prior to the start of the factor VIII protein-coding region, and the coding region itself, as well as the number of exons and introns contained within the gene. This type of information can eventually be useful in isolating, or possibly synthesizing, a normal DNA sequence for factor VIII that can then be used to correct this sequence defect through gene therapy.

Ultimately, researchers expect to sequence the genomes of individuals in order to figure out what makes us different. This type of rapid sequencing capability is needed, not just for sequencing human genomes, but also for animal and plant genomes, as well as for pathogenic microorganisms in the event of a germ warfare attack. We have already seen the application of DNA sequencing in the rapid identification of the strain of anthrax used in the 2001 bioterrorism attacks on the United States.

Genetic tools: DNA typing (DNA fingerprinting)   Restriction enzymes and DNA probes were key to developing the identification technology known as DNA typing, which is now used routinely in forensic laboratories. The purpose of DNA typing is to be able to distinguish one person from another and to be able to do so unequivocally. Here's how it works. Every individual is genetically different from every other individual, with the exception of genetically identical siblings. Every cell with a nucleus contains DNA, such as white blood cells, sperm, or cells from the hair bulb or the lining of the cheek. When DNA is collected from one of these sources and cut with a set of restriction enzymes, fragments are generated. The number of fragments produced and the length of each fragment will vary with the restriction enzyme used and with the individual. Each enzyme has a unique recognition site, the sequence of DNA bases where it can cut the DNA chain. Furthermore, each individual's DNA sequence is slightly different from any other individual's; thus the number of recognition sites for the restriction enzymes, as well as the number and length of fragments, will differ. These fragments can be separated from each other using a gel matrix and an electric current transferred to a solid support (such as a membrane or piece of filter paper) and treated with labeled

DNA probes to produce a visible pattern of fragments. This pattern is characteristic of an individual, and it can be used to identify that individual. DNA typing is now routinely used to identify victims at sites of airplane crashes, natural disasters, military engagements, and so on.

DNA typing has been admissible as evidence in criminal cases since the 1980s, and it is now routinely used as a tool in forensic laboratories to identify perpetrators or to clear an individual who has been falsely accused of, and sometimes imprisoned for, a crime of which that person is innocent. Sperm recovered from a rape victim can quickly identify the rapist. With modern DNA amplification techniques, the DNA recovered from a single cell can construct the genetic fingerprint of the perpetrator. Each of the states, under the leadership of the Federal Bureau of Investigation, participates in a national database that contains the genetic fingerprints of known perpetrators. See the information on minisatellites in the "Comparative Genomics" section for details about the specific sequences used for identification purposes.

This same basic approach can also be used to identify paternity, and it has been applied to human beings and animals. The mother and father will have characteristic genetic fingerprints when a sample of their DNA is cut with restriction enzymes. When the child's DNA is subjected to the same restriction enzymes and then run in the gel alongside those of the putative parents, each one of the child's DNA fragments will match one of the parents' fragments. In other words, the child's genetic fingerprint will clearly derive from those of the parents. In a recent parentage case, the descendants of Sally Hemings, a slave owned by Thomas Jefferson, were able to establish that they were also descended from Jefferson. Using genetic evidence carried on the Y chromosome, which is inherited virtually unchanged from father to son, modern-day genetic sleuths were able to detect genetic information from Jefferson's Y chromosome in the male descendants of Hemings, thereby establishing Jefferson as the male ancestor.

States routinely use DNA typing to identify the father when the child's mother seeks support payment from a man who denies parentage. Increasingly, DNA typing is being used to establish paternity in purebred animals, particularly in horses where large sums of money are involved. Sperm, rather than horses, is shipped around the world and used to impregnate mares. The opportunities for error or fraud are significant, making DNA typing especially useful in this business.

Genetic tools: transgenic organism technology   Recombinant DNA technology also led to the development of transgenic organism technology, the ability to transfer genetic material from one species to another to produce transgenic organisms. In plants, transgenic technology is used effectively for crop development. Generally the host plant has desirable characteristics, and the transferred gene confers an advantage or adds one or more desirable traits. The plants may be food crops for human beings or animals, or they may produce other usable products such as cotton, flax, or commercially desirable oils. The gene or genes transferred may make the plant hardier such that it becomes resistant to many of the forces of nature that diminish yield or, with food crops, nutritional value and marketability. Transgenic plants are also being developed for producing therapeutic molecules (see later section "Applications of Genetic Technology to Food Production").

In animals, transgenic technology is used to address environmental problems; to generate skin, hearts, kidneys, and other body parts for transplantation purposes; to construct model systems for use by researchers in answering complex genetic questions, or those such as in toxicology that are too dangerous to answer with human subjects; and to develop therapeutic proteins for clinical applications. An interesting example of an environmental application of transgenic animal technology is the Enviropig developed by Canadian scientists. This pig contains bacteria and mouse genes that make its manure less environmentally harmful than that of other pigs. Manure is heavy in phosphorus, and runoff from hog farms is a major cause of pollution in various bodies of water throughout North America. The transgenic Enviropig can digest the phosphorus in cereal feed much more efficiently than the standard pig, which reduces the environmental impact.

The main application of transgenic technology has been to develop model systems for laboratory studies intended to address complex basic research questions and to generate therapeutic proteins. Researchers routinely use model systems to provide an in vivo assay that mimics the human response as closely as possible. In vitro assays have provided invaluable insight into mechanisms of action, but they have no direct application to human biochemistry and physiology. Model systems offer the advantages of controlled breeding experiments and genetic manipulations. They permit the assessment of gene involvement in toxic chemical and cancer-causing reactions, and they enable experimentation such that the steps in these processes can be determined and interventions can be tried without the potential risk to human subjects.

Transgenic technology has been applied to several species such as cows, goats, sheep, pigs, rabbits, chickens, and fish, but by far the most widely used transgenic animal is the laboratory mouse. The gene to be transferred–the *transgene*–is carefully prepared to contain not only the coding region for the protein of interest but also all of the critical sequences involved in transcription in the tissue desired. Gene expression can occur in many tissues, or it can be confined to specific tissues, depending on the particular promoter region attached to the transgene. The transgene is introduced into the mouse genome by injection into fertilized eggs. DNA from the mouse pups is tested for the presence of the transgene, and then the particular tissue in which the transgene is to be expressed is tested to be certain that the transgene is expressed. Pups containing the transgene are called *founders*. After appropriate matings of the founders to establish a line in which the transgene is homozygous in each mouse, the transgenic line is ready for use.

Two fundamental questions that are asked using transgenic model systems are the effect of overexpression of a gene, which can be tested in an organism constructed to have multiple copies of a gene (multiple-copy organisms), and the effect of having no copies of a gene (*knockout organisms*). A mouse model system involving multiple copies of the beta amyloid protein precursor (the *APP* gene) was developed to study the role of this protein in Alzheimer's disease. When the transgene is incorporated into the mouse genome, one to two hundred copies are typically integrated in a head-to-tail orientation into a single random position in the mouse genome. The end result is multiple copies of a single gene, which yields an excess of the protein for which that gene codes. In this case, a mutant form of *APP* was transferred to mice, which results in the overproduction of an altered form of beta amyloid protein precursor. These animals developed neuropathological changes similar to those seen in Alzheimer's disease, which suggested a primary role for the *APP* gene in the development of this disorder.

The effect of diet on the development of Alzheimer's disease is also being tested using transgenic mice. Those fed a hypercholesterolemic diet were found to produce significantly higher levels of amyloid precursor protein. Having established transgenic animal model systems for Alzheimer's disease, it is now possible to test potential therapies for preventing or delaying its onset and, hopefully, to accelerate the search for answers to this debilitating disorder.

Similarly, transgenic mice can be used to study the effect of the absence of a gene. These mice are called knockout mice (or simply knockouts) and are increasingly useful as the research focus shifts to identifying the protein product of each gene and the function of these proteins. Just as multiple-copy mice can be examined for the effect of having too much of a protein, the effect of having too little of a protein can be examined using knockouts. One example of a knockout model is mice that have had their *IL-10* gene disrupted. This gene codes for the cytokine interleukin-10, a protein suspected of dampening the inflammatory response initiated by other cytokines. Knockout *IL-10* mice develop enterocolitis similar to Crohn's disease in human beings. Not only have these mice confirmed the suspected role of *IL-10* as an anti-inflammatory cytokine, they provide a model system for studying Crohn's disease, a painful gastrointestinal disorder that erodes the mucosal lining of the gut and can penetrate across the gut wall.

Both of these approaches are important to understanding the association between a gene and a disease. A new gene that links hypertriglyceridemia to increased risk of cardiovascular disease was discovered using transgenic mice (Pennachio et al. 2001). The gene *APOAV* was transferred to mice so that it was overexpressed. The same strain of mouse was also constructed to be a knockout devoid of *APOAV* activity. When plasma triglyceride levels were measured, those with extra copies of the gene had triglyceride levels one-third those of the controls, and those with no copies of the gene had levels four times those of the controls. These experiments suggest that the *APOAV* gene is important in maintaining normal triglyceride levels.

Beyond the laboratory applications of transgenic animal systems as model systems to study gene-function or gene-disease associations, transgenic animals are also used to produce therapeutic proteins. Initially recombinant therapeutic proteins were produced by genetically engineering bacteria because of their rapid growth rate. Many proteins continue to be made in this way, but not all proteins are expressed efficiently in lower organisms. Many proteins important to higher organisms such as mammals are glycosylated to become glycoproteins. Bacteria do not produce glycosylated proteins and thus do not provide an effective production system for many therapeutic proteins. Among the systems being developed to fill this void are transgenic animals, particularly cows, goats, and sheep, all of which produce milk. Human proteins can be integrated into the animal's genome, enabling the expressed proteins to be secreted in the milk and readily collected. This system is particularly useful for proteins required in high volume. Among the proteins produced in this way are therapeutic recombinant monoclonal antibodies used in cancer therapy, recombinant human serum albumin used as a blood-volume extender, and the recombinant therapeutic proteins antithrombin III, alpha$_1$ antitrypsin, and alpha glucosidase.

Comparative Genomics

The underlying basis for the identification technology mentioned earlier is genetic variation, not the gross morphological variation seen with changes in chromosome number or structure and affecting thousands of genes; rather, they are more subtle changes that cannot be readily seen and that must be detected at the molecular level. This type of variation may involve only a single DNA base change. In Chapter 3 we discussed the concept of mutation, the variation in genes that results over time, and its potential effect on function. A single base change in a gene can result in a change in the amino acid sequence of the protein and have devastating effects, as with sickle cell disease, or it may be silent if it falls within the noncoding region. The locus of a gene is polymorphic when there are two or more alleles occurring in at least one percent of the population studied. In other words, these alleles are common enough to be detected, given the right tools. Some polymorphic loci have only two alleles; others have multiple variations.

Detection of genetic variations of this nature requires a much finer resolution than is used to visualize chromosomes, and it takes advantage of natural variations such as *restriction fragment length polymorphisms, variable number of tandem repeats, microsatellites,* and *single nucleotide polymorphisms.* Each of these variations alters the normal DNA fragment pattern generated by restriction enzymes, and these altered patterns can be detected and used to distinguish one species from another as well as to detect individuals within a species. Technically, comparative genomics refers to comparisons between species. Comparing sequences within a species is called DNA sequence variation, but the basic principle is the same: comparing a sequence base for base to detect the extent of similarity (homology).

Detecting sequence variation by RFLPs   Restriction fragment length polymorphism (RFLP) was the first type of sequence variation to be used to detect genetic differences between individuals. These variations detect the presence or absence of a restriction site (i.e., the DNA base sequence that a particular restriction enzyme recognizes). In this case, a locus has only two alleles: it either has the correct DNA sequence that the restriction enzyme can recognize and cut, or it does not. If the DNA from two individuals is isolated and cut with the restriction enzyme *Eco*RI, for example, the enzyme will recognize the DNA sequence GAATTC and cut the DNA every place that sequence occurs. For simplicity, let's say there are normally four recognition sites for *Eco*RI within the human genome, which results in five DNA fragments. The number and length of these fragments can be characterized. If an individual has a mutation at one of these sites, the enzyme will not cut at that point, and only four fragments will be generated; the uncut fragment will be longer than any of the fragments generated normally. Using just this single enzyme, the two individuals can be distinguished by differences in their RFLP patterns. There are thousands of known restriction enzymes that can generate different RFLPs, thereby creating a system for detecting genetic variation among individuals.

Analysis of RFLPs can also be used to detect a genetic change associated with a disease and to help locate the gene for that disease on a chromosome. For example, RFLP analysis was helpful in locating the gene for the form of eye cancer known as retinoblastoma. By combining conventional chromosome staining with RFLP technology, the gene for retinoblastoma was discovered on chromosome 13. The disease was associated with a missing band (stained region) on the chromosome. Researchers then searched for retinoblastoma-associated RFLPs in that region of chromosome 13 and developed a detection assay for the disease.

Detecting sequence variation by VNTRs   The variable number of tandem repeats (VNTRs) is a variation on RFLPs. VNTRs contain multiple alleles, thereby providing more information about genetic diversity than RFLPs. These variations are regions of DNA scattered throughout the human genome that have the same DNA sequence repeated over and over. The repeat sequence is typically twenty to seventy base pairs long and occurs a variable number of times in different individuals; the multiple copies are arranged in tandem. These regions of repetitive DNA are called *minisatellites*.

Another type of repetitive DNA is the microsatellite, also called a *short tandem repeat* (STR). Like minisatellites, these regions occur in variable number and are arranged in tandem, but the repeat sequence is only two to six base pairs long. Technically microsatellites are not VNTRs but, from a practical standpoint, they can be thought of as a smaller type of VNTR, useful for the same purposes.

Both types of repetitive sequences are highly variable among individuals, which has made them useful for detecting genetic diversity, for identification purposes, and as markers for mapping genes to chromosomes. Their biological purpose, however, remains unknown. We do know that there are at least 100,000 microsatellites in the human genome and that they are associated with a variety of neurological diseases, which makes them useful as markers for detecting those at risk. Huntington's disease is the best studied of these neurological disorders. The normal gene, which codes for a large protein of unknown function, contains ten to thirty units of a tandemly arranged three-base repeat (a microsatellite) that codes for the amino acid glutamine such that multiple copies of this amino acid are inserted near the beginning of the protein. Individuals destined to develop Huntington's disease contain a microsatellite that codes for thirty-six or more glutamines. This disease is an autosomal-dominant disorder; thus, just one copy of the expanded repeat is sufficient to trigger the late-onset dementia and gradual loss of motor control that characterize the disease.

Microsatellites have also become useful markers for the early detection of cancer. In some cancers, such as colorectal and bladder cancer, the length of the microsatellite changes early on in the development of these cancers and provides an early warning signal for problems ahead.

Detecting sequence variation by SNPs   Additionally, there are sequence variations that involve a single nucleotide (DNA base) change, called single nucleotide polymorphisms (SNPs, pronounced "snips"). If we compared the DNA of two individuals base for base, there would be a difference in a single base for about every one to two hundred bases (Stephens et al., 2001). In a genome of three billion bases, that degree of difference adds up to a lot of variation and is the reason that two human beings, although at least 99.9 percent genetically homologous, look and act differently.

Single nucleotide polymorphisms, then, refer to the single base changes that occur at regular intervals throughout a genome and that are responsible for the slight variations among individuals. These variations are expected to be useful from a basic science standpoint as well as for health-related applications. Basic science interests include the amount of genetic variation among human beings and the significance of this variation. A major health-related issue is how to translate the understanding of this variation into improved health care.

To examine the degree of variation within the human population, DNA samples are sequenced from anonymous unrelated males and females whose genetic ancestry collectively represents the major populations of the world. The DNA sequence of each individual is compared base by base and the similarities and differences noted. Great care has been taken to ensure anonymity both of the individual donors and of the racial and ethnic groups represented in order to prevent potential stigmatization. Given these safeguards, the data cannot tell us how races or ethnic groups differ from one another, but they can provide insight into how uniform the human species is overall.

The health-related applications of SNPs are expected to be particularly useful. It is estimated that each human gene exists in twelve different versions on average. A major goal of the Human Genome Project is to associate such sequence variations with inheritable phenotypes such as particular disease conditions. By sequencing a large number of SNPs within coding regions of genes and correlating them with their impact on the function of the gene's protein product and the individual's phenotype (disease versus wellness), it will be possible to determine how each base in the DNA relates to the function of the product of that gene and to particular disease states.

One example of a clinical application of SNPs that is already in progress is the genetic profiling of individuals with respect to the genes that code for the major drug-metabolizing enzymes, such as the CYP 450 enzymes. These genes are polymorphic and result in the highly variable responses to drugs that patients experience. Another example is the anticipation that individuals who suffer from type 2 diabetes mellitus can be subdivided through SNP identification into those who can benefit from the thiazolidinediones and those who cannot. These polymorphisms are expected to provide a tie between particular base changes and particular drug responses, as well as to provide a way to generate genetic profiles of individuals with respect to each of the major drug-metabolizing genes. Once it can be determined which genotypes respond positively and which negatively to a drug, physicians can begin to tailor drug recommendations to the individual patient.

Genotype profiling via SNPs can also help to guide therapy by being able to distinguish among diseases that manifest similarly but that are actually distinct disorders requiring different therapeutic approaches. For example, a group of four cancer syndromes in children—neuroblastoma, rhabdomyosarcoma, non-Hodgkin's lymphoma, and the Ewing family of tumors—manifest identically but respond differently to treatment. Obviously, the physician's ability to distinguish among the four types may well make the difference between life and death for the child with one of these cancers.

Researchers also expect SNPs to be helpful in predicting susceptibility to disease and in dissecting the complexities of the chronic diseases such as cardiovascular disease, cancer, diabetes, psychiatric disorders, and the like. To do so will require researchers to obtain DNA from numerous disease-affected and disease-unaffected individuals, as well as to compare a large number of their SNPs to determine which are associated with the disease. Essentially, many thousands of SNPs spanning the entire human genome need to be identified, and an extensive database of DNA sequence information from individuals needs to be generated. Using computer matching of SNPs with the various disorders these individuals have, a specific SNP can be associated with a particular disorder and can serve as a marker for predicting susceptibility to that disorder. By identifying numerous SNPs, each specific to a particular disease, genotypic profiles can be developed that correlate to the degree of risk an individual has of developing each of the represented diseases.

Clearly, SNPs are regarded as a major tool for reducing genetic research to useful clinical applications. Before SNPs can become a commercial reality, however, much basic science involving the association of a given SNP with a particular effect, whether a disease condition or the ability to metabolize a drug, is necessary. Before SNPs reach their full potential for applications such as predicting disease susceptibility or drug response, research typically projected to last five to ten years must be carried out according to the following stages:

- The initial stage, basic research involving the discovery of new SNPs, requires screening a high volume of DNA sequences to identify the polymorphisms. (Roughly three million SNPs have already been identified, and the number increases regularly.) This stage is well underway.
- The next stage concerns validation of these SNPs in diverse populations, making sure that the sequences identified hold up as diagnostic across a number of populations. This stage, too, is underway.
- Next, large-scale association studies that will correlate specific SNPs with particular diseases or particular drug efficacies, tested in large population samples, will have to be conducted.
- Subsequently these SNPs will be used in clinical trials. The trial population may be selected based on genotype profiles. For example, the effect of a drug on a preselected genetic population may be studied, such as those at high risk for developing a particular disease or those who have the genetic makeup to metabolize a drug effectively with maximal benefit and minimal side effects.
- The final stage will be the widespread introduction of genotyping tools into clinical diagnostics.

Microarray technology   Ultimately the most direct method for determining genetic differences will be to sequence the individual's DNA. At this time, DNA sequencing is still too time-consuming and expensive to be used routinely. Other techniques that can rapidly discover mutations of health consequence are being developed. Chief among them is the *microarray*, also called the *DNA chip*. Microarrays provide a means of large-scale mutation detection because thousands of disease-causing mutations can be tested for in a single, rapid analysis, and the results can be analyzed by computer. They can, in effect, monitor the whole genome on a single chip, which provides a means of assessing the interaction of thousands of genes simultaneously.

The two major applications of microarrays are (1) to identify a DNA sequence, such as comparing the similarity between the DNA of two different organisms or testing whether a DNA sample contains a mutation compared with the normal version, and (2) to determine the level of expression of a gene, which can vary depending on the development stage of the organism and various environmental factors.

The microarray itself is a small glass plate much like a microscope slide, manufactured by a process similar to that used to make computer chips—hence the common name. The underlying basis for the assay is complementary base pairing (A with T, G with C). Single-stranded DNA sequences are spotted onto the plate. Each spot contains many copies of the same DNA sequence, and thousands of spots representing different DNA sequences can be placed on a single plate. Microarrays are versatile, and the DNA on the plate will differ depending on the purpose of the assay. If the human genome is compared to the fruit fly genome, for example, DNA fragments representing the entire human genome might be attached to the plate. Labeled DNA from the fruit fly genome would be allowed to interact with the DNA on the microarray plate, and the amount of fruit fly DNA that hybridizes (binds to the human DNA on the microarray plate through complementary base pairing) gives a good indication of the degree of genetic similarity between the two genomes.

Clinical applications of microarrays include diagnostic assays for mutations associated with diseases. For example, microarrays can be used to test a woman at high risk for breast cancer to see whether she has a mutation in the breast cancer gene *BRCA1*. In this case, normal *BRCA1* fragments are attached to the plate. A blood sample is obtained from the woman, the DNA is removed and cut into small single-stranded fragments, and it is then labeled with a colored fluorescent dye. If the woman does not have a mutation in *BRCA1*, her DNA will bind with the DNA on the microarray plate, and the fluorescence is readily detected. If she does have a mutation in *BRCA1*, her DNA will not hybridize in the region where the mutation is located. That region can then be examined more closely.

Microarrays also play an important role in distinguishing among different types of cancer that manifest identically but result from different mutations and require different therapeutic approaches. For example, women with breast cancer are offered specific therapies depending on their genetic expression profiles. Microarray analysis has been used to distinguish *BRCA1* and *BRCA2* breast cancer gene mutations and to show that they cause breast cancer through different molecular pathways, a finding that directly affects therapeutic options. Without microarray analysis, breast cancer drug therapy would still be hit-or-miss rather than a considered approach.

Cancer is not the only therapeutic application of microarray technology. Recently scientists generated genetic profiles for Crohn's disease and ulcerative colitis, two inflammatory bowel disorders that are difficult to distinguish, particularly in their early stages. Using microarray technology to screen over seven thousand genes, researchers were able to identify genes that were uniquely altered in Crohn's disease, in ulcerative colitis, or in both. This type of research paves the way for diagnostic tests that can assist with an accurate diagnosis early in the disease process.

In addition to comparing genomes between organisms and developing diagnostic assays, microarrays are useful for studying the process of gene expression and its regulation. They can be used to detect which genes are expressed in a cell, to compare gene expression patterns between two cell types such as liver and brain cells, to analyze cells from the same tissue to determine which genes are expressed at different times during development, and to determine the effect on gene expression when DNA is exposed to a variety of environmental factors.

Several clinical applications are already in use. Acute myeloid leukemia (AML) and acute lymphoblastic leukemia (ALL) are two cancers that are difficult to distinguish by conventional pathology, but that can be more easily distinguished by their different gene expression patterns using microarray technology. Similarly, the small, round, blue cell tumors of childhood cannot be subclassified into the four types of cancer that they represent using standard technology, but they can be distinguished based on the expression profiles generated by microarray analysis. This classification is critical because the four cancers require different therapeutic approaches. Likewise, with non-Hodgkin's lymphoma, microarray technology demonstrated that there were at least two subclasses of non-Hodgkin's lymphoma based on the genes expressed and that different therapies were appropriate for the two cancer types.

The microarray is an important technological advance for both basic research applications and clinical applications that range from detecting disease susceptibility to directing the choice of drugs and other therapeutic options. Another far-reaching potential role for microarrays is the ability to combine information from multiple genes to formulate a genotypic profile of an individual that can be used to predict virtually any gene-related activity, from the diseases for which that individual is at increased susceptibility to how well the individual is likely to respond to a particular drug or to digest and absorb a particular food. Each of these characteristics is ultimately rooted in the individual's genetic makeup; having a profile of that makeup provides insight into the functional ability of that individual.

MAPPING GENES TO CHROMOSOMAL LOCATIONS

Part of the quest of the Human Genome Project is to physically map each gene at a particular location on a particular chromosome. Mapping genes precedes the Human Genome Project by many decades, however, and was an early goal of geneticists. For basic research purposes, scientists wanted to be able to account for each gene, as well as to know where it was located and how close two genes were to each other. For plant and animal breeding, it was important to know the probability that two genes would stay together (a property of their being physically close together on a chromosome) and end up together in the offspring. In medical applications, the chromosome on which a gene is located and how close it is to another gene are important in calculating the risk that an individual will inherit a disease that runs in the family. For example, knowing that the gene for hemophilia A is recessive and is located on the X chromosome (from pedigree analysis of many families) allows for the prediction that all male offspring of hemophilia A mothers and non-hemophiliac fathers can be expected to have hemophilia A, and that all female offspring will be carriers.

There are different types of genetic maps. Linkage maps show the order and distance between genes and other DNA sequences whose inheritance can be followed (with markers) on a chromosome. Physical maps provide differing levels of detail about the structure of a chromosome, from increasingly detailed positioning information about the gene or marker to the actual base sequence. Mapping a chromosome means positioning genes or markers on a chromosome in the correct order and at the distance from neighboring genes or markers, and ultimately determining the base sequence from one end of the chromosome to the other.

Chromosome mapping makes use of both linkage maps and physical maps. First the mode of inheritance of a gene or marker is determined, which indicates whether the sequence is found on one of the sex chromosomes or on an autosome; it also indicates its proximity to any other marker that has already been assigned a chromosomal location. This information does not, however, tell you on which chromosome the gene or marker is found. To place a marker on a specific chromosome, either linkage analysis or DNA probe analysis can be used.

The basis of linkage analysis is that two DNA segments physically close to each other on a chromosome will tend to be inherited together. During meiosis, the process by which sperm and egg cells are formed, the forty-six chromosomes find their mates (called homologous chromosomes or *homologues*) and actually pair along their length. During this unique pairing, physical exchange of chromosomal material occurs between the homologues. Since each homologue has the same basic genetic configuration but differs slightly in its DNA base sequences (one homologue comes from the mother, the other from the father), swapping pieces of chromosomes results in new genetic combinations in the sperm and egg cells.

In a mating in which two genes or markers on a particular chromosome are followed, the closer the genes are to each other, the less the chance that an exchange will occur between them and separate them. They would tend to stay together and be inherited together in the offspring. The farther apart they are, the more likely an exchange would occur, and the two genes would end up separated into different sperm or egg cells. In other words, genetic linkage can be determined by how frequently two markers are passed together from parent to child. By counting the number of offspring with both genes and the number with just one of the two genes, one can calculate the distance between the two genes. Similarly, by using three genes, both the distance between any two pairs and the order of the three genes can be determined by measuring outcomes in the offspring.

If the map is sufficiently detailed that several other markers have already been positioned on each of the chromosomes, linkage to a marker places the gene on the same chromosome as the marker. If linkage to a known marker cannot be demonstrated, DNA probes can be used to figure out which chromosome the gene is on. A probe is made from the gene's DNA sequence; it is tagged with an indicator such as radioactivity or fluorescent color and incubated with a set of chromosomes. The probe will bind to the chromosome where the gene is located, much like two pieces of Velcro finding and sticking to each other. The tag allows the probe to be visualized so that, in addition to identifying which chromosome the gene is on, the probe indicates the location of the gene along the chromosome.

On linkage maps, distances between markers are measured in *centimorgans* (cM), a unit named after the American geneticist Thomas Hunt

Morgan. A distance of 1 cM is equal to one percent recombination, meaning that two linked genes are separated in the offspring only one percent of the time. Distances between markers in physical maps are measured in the number of bases. A genetic distance of 1 cM is equal to a physical distance of 1 million DNA bases.

To learn more about a chromosome itself, one can use physical maps of increasing resolution. First, numerous copies of a single human chromosome are isolated. Using rDNA techniques, the chromosome is broken down into overlapping fragments by using restriction enzymes that cut the chromosome in different places. The number of copies of each fragment is amplified, either by cloning or by PCR, and then physically separated by gel electrophoresis. Researchers look for recognizable markers among the fragments and, much like assembling a jigsaw puzzle, seek fragments that share markers, to begin the tedious process of reassembling the chromosome. Fortunately, technological advances now permit computers to take the overlapping fragments and reconstruct the original chromosome. Once the order of the fragments has been established, the final step is to determine the actual DNA sequence for each fragment, and ultimately for the entire chromosome. Developing automated processes and computer programs to replace the required manual labor and greatly speeding up this process is one of the many contributions the Human Genome Project is making to genetic research.

Although the ultimate information is the DNA base sequence of the entire chromosome, and a physical map would seem to be far superior to a linkage map, linkage maps still play a valuable role in determining a gene's location and the distance between that gene and a known marker. Linkage maps are particularly valuable for associating diseases with specific genes or markers. The gene itself or its protein product may not yet be identified; however, by finding that it shows linkage to particular markers, the chromosomal location for the gene that causes the disease can be pinpointed. Once that chromosomal location is known, the gene's inheritance pattern and probability of being inherited in the offspring can be predicted. This information often leads to an early diagnostic test; the marker linked to the gene serves as the basis for this test. Examples of diseases originally mapped this way include sickle cell disease, Tay-Sachs disease, cystic fibrosis, myotonic dystrophy, and fragile X syndrome. The current status of the mapping of human disease genes can be viewed at a Web page titled OMIM: The Online Mendelian Inheritance of Man (see "Useful Web Resources" section).

The main purpose of gene mapping is easily lost in all the details. Mapping genes is expected to help us understand the biological basis of disease. The first step is to associate a disease with the chromosome and then to narrow that association to a particular region of the chromosome and, ultimately, to a specific gene within that region. Once a gene has been located, it can be cloned and its DNA sequence determined. This sequence can then be expressed and the protein identified. The protein's normal structure and function can be studied, and changes in that structure and function can be identified and correlated with changes in the DNA sequence. This collective information pinpoints the molecular basis for the disease and provides the information necessary for both drug and gene therapy approaches.

Obviously, human beings do not lend themselves readily to controlled mating experiments. Fortunately, progress with the human map has been greatly accelerated by the use of model organisms such as those discussed earlier. Many of the so-called housekeeping genes of living organisms are the same. Model organisms such as yeast and other microorganisms, the roundworm, the fruit fly, and the laboratory mouse have many of the same genes as human beings, and they can be manipulated genetically. Strains are developed that contain the desired genetic background into which a new gene can be introduced. The gene's location and distance on a chromosome relative to known markers can be calculated. Mutations can be introduced, and the effects of these mutations on function can be observed, such as the multiple-copy and knockout systems discussed earlier. Just generating the large quantity of offspring necessary for these types of experiments has been a major contribution of model systems.

FUNCTIONAL GENOMICS: DISCOVERING THE IDENTITY AND FUNCTION OF EACH GENE PRODUCT

Whereas the initial phase of the Human Genome Project focused on gene discovery, the focus now is on the so-called functional genomics. This research emphasis concerns linking a function to each discovered gene and ultimately linking disease to the dysfunction of genes and their protein products. Since the production of proteins is under the control of the intricate regulatory networks that regulate the expression of genes, functional genomics also concerns the function of the noncoding regions of the genome and of the large number of SNPs that exist throughout the human genome in both the coding and noncoding regions. The subspecialty area of functional genomics, proteomics, focuses on identifying the proteins themselves and their role in the functioning of living organisms.

In biology, the whole is much greater than the sum of its parts. Having the sequences of millions of pieces of DNA has been likened to having all the parts of a car without having insight into the complex workings of the assembled car. Similarly, DNA sequences do not provide information as to how those sequences work together to create a living organism. What is required is a set of technological tools that moves beyond identifying DNA sequences to identifying the protein products of each coding sequence, their functions in the organism, and the consequences of errors in the genetic material that lead to dysfunctional proteins. Two technological developments have been key to the progress made in functional genomics thus far: model systems and microarrays.

The Mouse Model System in Functional Genomics

Functional genomics is studied using the laboratory mouse as a primary model system. As discussed earlier, model systems have been essential to the progress of genetic research. They can be genetically manipulated at the molecular level and offer a cost-effective way to study genes and their effects over a number of generations in a relatively short period of time. Mice are used because they are genetically quite similar to human beings. Although the extent of similarity will not be known for certain until both genomes are completely and accurately sequenced, it is suspected that ninety-nine percent of human genes have a mouse counterpart. From the DNA databases being developed from the sequencing data from the human and mouse genome sequencing projects, it is possible to identify a gene in human beings and locate the counterpart in the mouse. The knockout mouse is particularly useful because when a new human gene is discovered, its mouse counterpart gene can be identified and mutated, or knocked out, and the effect of the lack of this gene's function on the health of the mouse can be observed. By extrapolation, these observations in the mouse are applied to human beings with striking success.

Earlier we discussed the use of the *IL-10* knockout mouse to assign an anti-inflammatory role to the cytokine protein interleukin-10 and to provide a model system for studying the inflammatory bowel disorder Crohn's disease. Another example of a knockout system comes from the surprise development of a mouse model for studying obesity. Researchers developed a knockout mouse in which the gene that codes for the protein pro-opiomelanocortin (POMC) was incapacitated. POMC is a precursor for a number of neurotransmitters and hormones, including the alpha melanocyte–stimulating hormone responsible for pigmentation. The original plans for this model system were to study neuropeptide signaling during the development of the central nervous system. Instead, the mice were extremely obese and had yellowish fur as well as virtually no adrenal tissue. At about this time, German scientists reported studies with two children who had mutations in the *Pomc* gene. These children developed severe obesity within the first few months of life, adrenal insufficiency, and red hair. This mouse knockout model system will be useful for investigating the mechanism by which dysfunction in the *Pomc* gene leads to obesity, and it can also be used to test various approaches to intervention.

The above examples involve only a single gene. Genes and proteins are suspected of interacting in complex ways that multiply the functions of each, but we have so far lacked the technological tools for sorting out which gene is responsible for which actions. The mouse model system is expected to be helpful in this regard because strains can be constructed in which the effect of knocking out a single gene can be studied, and then these mice can be bred to create strains with more than one gene knocked out to study the collective effects of multiple genes and their products.

Microarrays in Functional Genomics

Microarray technology is used to ask questions about which genes are expressed, when they are expressed, and how they respond to various signals. The expression pattern of a gene is closely correlated to its biological role, so knowing in which tissues genes are expressed and which cellular and environmental signals turn a gene's expression on and off is expected to provide detailed clues to gene function.

For example, part of the mystery of human life is the developmental process whereby a single fertilized egg becomes a multicellular organism with cells that contain a complete set of genetic information but only express certain parts of that information. Furthermore, expression can change during the different stages of the developmental process. Microarray technology enables the researcher to ask which genes are expressed at each stage of development. This type of information is the first step in understanding which genes are critical and what each gene does. Having identified a key human gene, its mouse counterpart can be identified and knocked out so that a mouse strain is developed in which it is possible to examine the role of that particular gene in development. Mice that lack a functional version of this gene will likely have their development arrested. At which stage does this arrest take place and what are the consequences?

Tissue microarrays are used to detect which genes are expressed in which tissues in the body. Expression information is also important in determining the difference between a cancer cell and a normal cell, which affects therapeutic options, as will be seen in the next chapter on genetics and medical therapy. Microarrays are versatile and are expected to be a major tool for determining the roles of genes in the larger scheme of how an organism functions.

UNDERSTANDING THE REGULATION OF GENE EXPRESSION

Clearly, there is much to learn about the regulation of gene expression, and microarray technology provides the technical framework for asking complex questions about how genes are turned on and off and what regulates that expression. Several fundamental questions about cell function and response to the environment are being investigated using human cell lines and animal model systems.

One question concerns the differentiation of the various cell types that exist in higher organisms. A fundamental principle of biology is that all nucleated cells have the same DNA, but by selectively expressing certain genes, these cells can differentiate into cell types that are physically and functionally distinct. Bone cells are distinct from nerve cells, white blood cells, heart cells, and so on. How this selective control is accomplished is not yet known, but we do know it occurs. We see the results of dysfunctional control all the time: cancer resulting from abnormalities in the expression of genes involving cell growth and differentiation, metabolic disorders, hormone imbalances, or slow wound healing because of defects in the genetic signals controlling tissue regeneration.

Another key question concerns how gene expression differs between normal cells and cancer cells, and how that expression is influenced by various toxic chemicals and nutrients. Studies have begun to investigate diets such as those with high degrees of carbohydrate or fat consumption and their effects on gene expression. In each of these studies, microarray technology has been a prime tool.

Gene expression can potentially be regulated at any point along the pathway from DNA to protein, but transcriptional regulation is the primary mode of regulation in higher organisms and is the main focus of current research. Transcription factors are thought to be important players in regulating gene expression. These are a class of proteins that can turn gene expression on and off by interacting with the DNA in ways that promote or inhibit transcription. The details of transcriptional regulation in human beings are complex, potentially involving multiple locations in the gene, multiple transcription factors, and differences between cell types.

In vitro transcription assays are used to study the factors affecting gene expression. Single-stranded DNA is immobilized and incubated with the basic components needed to transcribe the DNA: RNA polymerase, nucleotides, and uridine that has been tagged (such as with radioactivity). Factors suspected of regulating gene expression are added, and the effect on mRNA production is measured.

Of significance to nutrition professionals is the fact that nutrients can bind to transcription factors and influence the action of these proteins in turning on and off gene expression, which suggests linkage among environmental signals and genetic material, and the potential for diet to influence gene expression. One example of a question concerning nutrient influence on gene expression is the responsiveness to cholesterol of the gene that codes for the low-density lipoprotein cholesterol (LDL-C) receptor. This receptor is on the surface of liver cells and binds to plasma LDL-C to facilitate its entry into liver cells. When cholesterol levels are high, the transcription of this gene is decreased because of an abundance of available cholesterol, and a normal level of transport into liver cells is sufficient to provide for cholesterol needs. When cholesterol levels are low, however, transcription is increased in order to enhance the ability to move cholesterol into the liver cell. What is not yet clear is the sequence of events that begins with cholesterol binding at the cell surface receptor and ends with unknown factors interacting with the DNA to enhance transcription of the LDL-C receptor gene.

Transgenic mice are expected to be useful in sorting out the steps and molecules in this sequence of events. Such mice have already been used to verify the gene and its function. Mice in which the LDL-C receptor gene is overexpressed show a significantly increased clearance of LDL-C from the blood. Knockout mice that cannot produce LDL-C receptors have abnormally high blood cholesterol levels. The types of experiments anticipated involve the ability to introduce mutations in different positions in the LDL-C receptor gene and to observe the effects on gene expression. Must there be an intact receptor in order to transmit the environmental signal that blood cholesterol levels are high and that increased transcription is needed to produce more LDL-C receptors? Does cholesterol interact directly with transcription factors, or with the DNA, or is there a chain of events set in motion by the binding of cholesterol to the receptor at the cell membrane? What makes the liver cell unique in its expression of LDL-C receptors? These types of gene-nutrient interaction questions can be asked using genetic technologies such as transgenic model systems and microarrays.

MONOCLONAL ANTIBODY TECHNOLOGY

A second major biotechnology in addition to recombinant DNA technology is *monoclonal antibody technology.* Monoclonal antibody production involves *hybridomas,* hybrid cells formed by fusing antibody-producing white blood cells and myeloma tumor cells. These hybrid cells can be grown in culture medium and have both the monoclonal antibody–producing properties of the white blood cells and the immortality of the tumor cells. The *mono-* refers to the ability to produce a single type of antibody, and *clonal* refers to the immortal cell line of identical cells (a clone), a significant step forward in the ability to produce human antibodies.

Antibody production is a normal part of the immune defense system of higher organisms. These proteins are produced by white blood cells in response to foreign proteins. Prior to monoclonal technology, antibodies were made by injecting animals such as rabbits and primates with foreign proteins, allowing several weeks or months for antibodies to be produced, and then obtaining them by collecting serum from the animal. This form of preparation, however, was actually polyclonal–a mixture of many monoclonal antibodies, each specifically recognizing a different part of the protein molecule. The individual monoclonal antibodies could not be separated from the mixture. Furthermore, the only source of additional antibody preparation was from the immunized animal, and when the animal died, the antibody supply died with it. In order to have more antibodies against that protein, another animal had to be immunized, and the antibody preparation that resulted was again polyclonal and could be quite different from the original preparation. Advances in biotechnology contributed the techniques of cell culture and cell fusion, enabling production of immortal cell lines that produced a never-ending supply of a single antibody with a single recognition site for the protein of interest.

Why is having an endless supply of a specific monoclonal antibody useful? The true asset of a monoclonal, as opposed to a polyclonal, antibody is its specificity for a limited region of a molecule or the cell surface of an organism. Such specificity is an asset when developing drugs; antibodies react with a specific target rather than with multiple targets, which often brings unintended side effects. An example of a monoclonal antibody–based pharmaceutical that capitalizes on site specificity is the monoclonal infliximab (Remicade) used for chronic inflammatory disorders such as Crohn's disease and ulcerative colitis. In this case the monoclonal prevents the pro-inflammatory cytokine molecule from binding to its cell surface receptor and initiating the cascade of events that leads to inflammation.

Monoclonal antibodies are also used as diagnostic reagents. The popular home pregnancy test kit is based on the ability of a monoclonal antibody to recognize beta human chorionic gonadotrophin (beta HCG), a molecule produced during early pregnancy. Monoclonals are used to screen blood samples and foods for undesirable agents such as infectious microorganisms. Another application of monoclonals, sound in principle but difficult to execute in practice, involves creating antibodies against unique proteins on the surface of cancer cells and attaching toxic chemicals to these specific antibodies to turn the monoclonal into a therapeutic agent that can target cancer cells and kill them. Such specificity would not be possible with a polyclonal antibody, which would react with normal cells as well as with cancer cells, rendering such an approach inappropriate as a cancer therapy. Once such useful applications are developed, it is essential that there be a reproducible method of generating additional antibodies with the same specificity. Such conditions could not be met with a traditional polyclonal antibody preparation, but are characteristic of monoclonal antibodies.

Monoclonal antibody formation is an evolving technology and it has been more difficult to perfect than was initially anticipated. The hybridoma cell lines can be finicky to grow and require a sort of laboratory green thumb to develop stable cultures that produce high levels of antibodies. As with any new technology, there are always issues to resolve, and monoclonal antibody production is no exception. Already there are a number of useful therapeutics on the market, and many more are anticipated over the next decade.

APPLICATIONS OF GENETIC TECHNOLOGY TO FOOD PRODUCTION

From the beginnings of agriculture, farmers have sought to breed plants and animals that were the highest-yield producers at the lowest cost, and that were the most resistant to disease. Until recently, making improvements to food animals and plants through conventional breeding programs was labor-intensive and time-consuming. Many reproductive cycles were required, and the process of obtaining the assortment of desired genes with a minimum of undesirable genes was mostly one of trial and error.

Development of recombinant DNA as well as transgenic plants and animals greatly improved the efficiency with which genetic applications could be used for breeding programs, and it generated new possibilities for the types of foods that could be produced. In addition to accelerated breeding programs, where only a limited portion of genetic material is transferred, major applications of genetic research include genetically engineering plants to increase yield, improving nutrition, expanding food production options, and producing therapeutic proteins; developing food safety detection systems; and genetically engineering animal food crops to improve yield and nutritional composition as well as produce therapeutic proteins.

Genetically Engineered Plant Food Crops

Plant crops have been genetically engineered with the primary goals of increasing crop yield and enhancing nutritional composition, but this technology can also expand food production options and produce therapeutic proteins in plants. Among the primary successes has been the ability to increase yield by developing plants that can withstand some of nature's more serious onslaughts.

Increase yield   Numerous plants have been genetically engineered to make them resistant to insects or better able to withstand harsh environmental conditions. Among these new varieties generated through pest resistance engineering are the following:

- Insect-protected cotton, corn, potatoes, tomatoes, canola, rice, apples, soybeans, and walnuts
- Virus-protected cantaloupe, papaya, squash, tomatoes, corn, potatoes, and alfalfa
- Insect- and virus-protected potatoes
- Bacterial-resistant potatoes
- Herbicide-tolerant soybeans, corn, cotton, canola, tomatoes, alfalfa, and potatoes

Attempts to improve environmental hardiness include:

- Drought-resistant canola, soybeans, corn, wheat, barley, and potatoes
- Cold-resistant tomatoes, strawberries, and potatoes
- Heat-resistant plants
- Plants that can grow in soils with high mineral and salt concentrations

An interesting approach to increasing man's control over the environment is the development of so-called sentinel plants, such as genetically engineered potatoes that would glow when the crop needed fertilizer, water, or additional pesticide or herbicide. These plants are not meant to be eaten but would be planted along with the food crop as a means of improving the yield (estimated at a threefold increase for potatoes) by alerting farmers to the need for water and food and potentially decreasing the use of fertilizer, pesticides, and herbicides.

Enhance nutritional composition   The need for foods enriched in the basic macronutrients or in health-protective components has fueled the drive to improve the nutritional composition of many crops:

- Amino acid–enhanced sweet potatoes, corn, soybeans, rice, and sunflowers
- Plants with an enhanced vitamin profile: rice with beta carotene; increased vitamin E in staple crops; increased provitamin A or lycopene content in tomatoes; higher levels of vitamins C and E in squash, tomatoes, and potatoes; and increased carotenoids in several plants
- Enhanced mineral nutrition in rice with increased iron content or corn strains that are low in phytic acid, a substance that can decrease mineral absorption
- Enhanced fatty acid profile: high-oleic acid soybeans, high-lauric acid canola oil, and high-stearate vegetable oils that can potentially decrease *trans* fatty acid content of foods by replacing hydrogenated oils
- Several plants with an enhanced phytonutrient profile: carrots with increased antioxidant beta carotene and anthocyanin content or rich in lycopene, onions and garlic containing anticlotting compounds, canola oil high in beta carotene, chicory with increased prebiotic inulin, and increased flavonol content in tomato peel

Changes in other characteristics of plants can potentially improve nutritional composition as well, such as increasing the solids content of tomatoes and potatoes, changing the carbohydrate content of potatoes to include increased starch and decreased simple sugars, and improving the postharvest properties of food, such as delayed ripening, improved chill tolerance, and controlled plant senescence. Enhancing the aesthetics of produce with improved color and flavor are other attempts to increase the consumption of fruits and vegetables.

Expand food production options   One of the fundamental goals of genetically engineering plants is to be able to feed the world as the global population expands and the amount of arable land available for farming shrinks. Genetic engineering is applied to expand our food options. One approach is producing genetically engineered marine foods and food-processing products (e.g., agarose, agar, and carageenan) by cultivating seaweed. Shrimp, snow crabs, and other crustacea grown in aquaculture are also being genetically engineered to increase fertility and hatchability.

Produce therapeutic proteins   Plants are also being genetically engineered to produce proteins that have therapeutic value to human beings and animals. Edible vaccines are a promising application. In this application, foods carry a vaccine that is harmless to human beings but that stimulates the immune system to make natural antibodies against a number of infectious organisms. Examples include potatoes and tomatoes engineered to contain an inactive hepatitis B virus, bananas and tomatoes containing genes that can help immunize against cholera, potatoes that protect against *E. coli*-related traveler's diarrhea, and bananas that carry a vaccine against the Norwalk virus. Edible vaccines against tetanus, whooping cough, and diphtheria are also of interest.

Another approach uses plants to make monoclonal antibodies, or "plantibodies," as they are called. The corn plant plays a key role here: it's the largest crop worldwide, and it naturally stores plantibodies in a low-moisture environment with a number of protective protease inhibitors, which help to preserve the antibody proteins. Producing monoclonal antibodies by traditional fermentation methods has been costly and fraught with technical problems. The plantibody approach may surmount some of the technical problems, and it may cost twenty-five to one hundred times less than traditional production methods.

One plantibody success so far is the production of fully human secretory IgA antibodies, a feat no other transgenic organism has yet mastered. Secretory IgA (sIgA) protects the mucosal surfaces of the eyes, nose, mouth, digestive tract, respiratory tract, and urogenital system from infection. The sIgA plantibodies inhibit *Streptococcus mutans*, the bacterium responsible for tooth decay, from binding to tooth surfaces and appear to prevent tooth decay for several weeks after application.

Many other therapeutic or industrially important proteins are being investigated for their production in plants, such as plantibodies against herpes simplex I and II, antisperm plantibodies to prevent conception, clot-dissolving drugs, hemoglobin, and virtually any pharmaceutically or industrially valuable protein.

Genetically Engineered Animal Food Crops

As with plants, the primary goals of genetically engineered animal crops are to increase yield and to enhance nutritional composition. These manipulations of the food supply have not been without controversy. Chapter 8 includes a discussion of policy issues relating to the food applications of biotechnology.

Increase yield   Recombinant bovine somatotropin (growth hormone, rBGH) has been used to increase milk production in cows. Recombinant porcine somatotropin is used to produce pork higher in lean muscle tissue and lower in fat. Other approaches are directed toward improving the fat composition of animal meat to make it more heart healthy.

Improved animal health essentially parallels the applications of biotechnology to human health: the use of recombinant DNA vaccines, monoclonal antibodies, immunomodulators, DNA diagnostic assays, and therapeutic proteins. Additionally, embryo cloning is used to make multiple copies of genetically valuable food animals and to increase yield. For example, the ability to preselect the sex of female chickens (laying hens) has a large economic impact.

One last application of genetic technology to food production concerns using DNA diagnostic assays for food and water safety–related applications. DNA probe assays have been developed to detect contaminants such as *Campylobacter, Listeria, Salmonella,* and *E. coli* 017:H57. These assays are rapid and highly specific.

APPLICATIONS OF GENETIC TECHNOLOGY TO HEALTH CARE

Among the expanded capabilities that rDNA technology brought to biotechnology are the ability to develop diagnostic tests for detecting existing disease and predicting susceptibility to future disease, diagnostic tests for food safety applications, the ability to synthesize proteins and vaccines that have therapeutic application in human beings and animals, and the potential for gene therapy, whereby genetic mutations can be corrected.

Diagnostic Testing

The clinical laboratory has benefited substantially from the development of a large number of DNA and RNA probe–based tests directed against infectious pathogens such as cytomegalovirus, the various hepatitis viruses, the herpes simplex viruses, Epstein-Barr virus, HIV, human papilloma virus, and numerous infectious bacteria, fungi, protozoa, and other parasites. The use of DNA probes to detect an individual's response to various drugs will soon become another major activity of the clinical lab and will, ultimately, move on to physicians' offices.

DNA probe tests have also been successfully applied to disease detection. There are literally thousands of assays now. Among the early successes are probes for the detection of cystic fibrosis, severe combined immunodeficiency disease (SCID), Huntington's, Duchenne's muscular dystrophy, Tay-Sachs disease, retinoblastoma, osteosarcoma, melanoma, the thalassemias, sickle cell disease, and hemophilia. Monoclonal antibody–based testing has been on the market for almost two decades and includes such in-home tests as ovulation and pregnancy detection.

Therapeutic proteins

One of the early applications of recombinant DNA technology was the production of therapeutic proteins such as the hormone insulin, and human growth hormone. To accomplish this, the segment of human DNA containing the insulin-producing gene is removed using restriction enzymes and spliced into the DNA of a bacterium. This unicellular organism grows in a simple broth and divides rapidly to form large numbers of identical bacteria. Each time a bacterium divides, it copies the human insulin gene contained in its genetic material. Each time a bacterium expresses its DNA, human insulin is made. This genetically engineered bacterium can be reproduced in large quantities, and the insulin it produces can be retrieved from the growth medium and used to treat people with diabetes, who can no longer make their own insulin. Numerous other therapeutic proteins can be made using this basic approach and will be discussed in the next chapter. Among them are human growth hormone, clotting factor VIII for treating hemophilia, interferons, interleukins, and various growth factors. Therapeutic proteins are also generated for use in veterinary medicine.

Therapeutic Organisms

A new type of therapeutic is on the horizon: the use of genetically engineered bacteria as probiotics that deliver a beneficial effect beyond that of probiotics alone. Probiotics are the friendly microorganisms that normally inhabit the gut and are instrumental in keeping gut tissue healthy and the functions of the digestive mucosa intact. When the mucosa becomes inflamed, which is seen in such gastrointestinal disorders as irritable bowel syndrome, Crohn's disease, ulcerative colitis, and the gluten-sensitive enteropathies, significant digestive dysfunction results. Bacteria can be engineered to secrete cytokines, such as IL-10, that have an anti-inflammatory effect on inflamed intestinal mucosa.

Vaccines

Recombinant DNA and monoclonal antibody technologies play a primary role in the development of vaccines for both human beings and animals. Early successes in human vaccine development include the hepatitis B and pertussis (whooping cough) vaccines. Animal vaccines include those against foot-and-mouth disease, porcine respiratory and reproductive syndrome, feline leukemia virus, and canine parvo virus. Biotechnology was the key to developing vaccines that protect animals against rabies and that protect cattle from the so-called shipping fever, a major killer of beef cattle in feedlots.

Gene Therapy

Similar techniques can be used for gene therapy. The DNA containing the faulty gene is isolated from human cells. The faulty gene is removed, a normal gene inserted, and the cells are then returned to the individual to multiply and produce the normal gene product. Gene replacement may involve somatic or germ line cells. Replacing a faulty gene with a normal gene in somatic cells involves bone marrow or other stem cell replacement. Such a change would correct the error in that individual but would not be inherited unless the gene was also replaced in the individual's germ line (sperm or egg) cells. When the error is corrected in the germ line, then the correction could be inherited. There is considerable controversy as to whether germ line gene therapy should take place. At present, only somatic cell gene therapy is permitted in the United States.

Somatic cell gene therapy is still a primitive process. The greatest chance for success at this point is to insert a normal gene for a recessive disorder that results from a nonfunctional or missing gene product, so that the normal gene can then supply the functional product. Often only a small level of the normal activity is needed to provide for the body's needs.

Many technological advances had to occur in order for gene therapy to be a possibility. In addition to the ability to associate a gene with a disease, locate that gene on the chromosome, isolate the gene, and amplify it, there has to be a way to introduce the gene into the tissue that needs its expression and have it copied and expressed by the cells of that tissue. Typically a virus is used as the vector. Viruses have evolved clever methods for getting their DNA into the cells they infect. They then commandeer the DNA copying process of the host so that the host makes new copies of the virus. The normal gene for the disease to be corrected is incorporated into the viral genome. When the virus enters the cell, the normal gene enters along with it and, when the cells begin to make virus DNA and protein, they also make the normal gene and its protein and provide the body with the missing protein. Developing effective vectors has held up the development of gene therapy, but the difficulties are technical and are expected to be overcome in time.

SOCIETAL CONCERNS ABOUT RECOMBINANT DNA TECHNOLOGY

The ability to use recombinant DNA technology to produce hybrid organisms that are new to nature is, understandably, of concern to society. In the same way the Human Genome Project integrated ethical, legal, and social issues into the project from the beginning, the scientific community has taken seriously the potential of rDNA technology for misuse and negative environmental impact. Since this technology began to be introduced in the early 1970s, prominent scientists have gathered on a regular basis to discuss the negative potential and to devise stringent guidelines that would minimize the possibility of harm. Beginning in 1975, conferences were held at Asilomar, California, and have therefore come to be known as the Asilomar Conferences. The initial concerns focused on the possibility of the infection of human beings with recombinant organisms or for the escape of these organisms into the wild, where they would be hard to control. Elaborate and costly containment protocols and facilities were developed to protect against these potential hazards. Luckily, these fears have been groundless to date. Over the years, as the safety of rDNA technology experiments has been continually demonstrated, the stringent precautions have been relaxed where possible. For those experiments that involve releasing recombinant DNA into the environment, as with agriculturally important plants, considerable caution is still recommended. Although not without controversy in the public arena, the scientific community is largely in agreement that rDNA technology is used responsibly and in ways that will benefit the environment and its many inhabitants. As with most if not all technological advances of our time, multigenerational experiments spanning many different experimental variations have not been performed prior to the broad-scale application of rDNA technology to medicine and food production. Despite the prognosis of some of the best minds within the scientific community, there are no guarantees that rDNA technology is safe in the long term.

Useful Resources

Collins FS, Brooks LD, Chakravarti A. A DNA polymorphism discovery resource for research on human genetic variation. *Genome Res.* 1998; 8:1229–1231.

Eisen MG, Brown PO. DNA arrays for analysis of gene expression. *Methods Enzymol.* 1999; 303:179–205.

Ekins R, Chu FW. Microarrays: their origins and applications. *Trends Biotechnol.* 1999; 17:217–218.

Hedenfalk I, Duggan D, Chen Y, et al. Gene-expression profiles in hereditary breast cancer. *N Engl J Med.* 2001; 344:539–548.

The International SNP Map Working Group. A map of human genome sequence variation containing 1.42 million single nucleotide polymorphisms. *Nature.* 2001; 409:928–933.

Khan J, Wei JS, Ringnér M, Saal LH, et al. Classification and diagnostic prediction of cancers using gene expression profiling and artificial neural networks. *Nat Med.* 2001; 7:673–679.

Mendoza C, Viteri FE, Lönnerdal B, Young KA, Raboy V, Brown KH. Effect of genetically modified, low-phytic acid maize on absorption of iron from tortillas. *Am J Clin Nutr.* 1998; 68:1123–1127.

Moxon ER, Wills C. DNA microsatellites: agents of evolution? *Sci Amer.* 1999; 1:94–99.

Pennacchio LA, Olivier M, Hubacek JA, et al. An apolipoprotein influencing triglycerides in humans and mice revealed by comparative sequencing. *Science.* 2001; 294:169–173.

Refolo LM, Malester B, LaFrancois J, et al. Hypercholesterolemia accelerates the Alzheimer's amyloid pathology in a transgenic mouse model. *Neurobiol Dis.* 2000; 7:321–331.

Shoemaker DD, Schadt EE, Armour CD, et al. Experimental annotation of the human genome using microarray technology. *Nature.* 2001; 409:922–927.

Song F, Srinivasan M, Aalinkeel R, Patel MS. Use of a cDNA array for the identification of genes induced in islets of suckling rats by a high-carbohydrate nutritional intervention. *Diabetes.* 2001; 50:2053–2060.

Stephens JC, Schneider JA, Tanguay DA, et al. Haplotype variation and linkage disequilibrium in 313 human genes. *Science.* 2001; 293:489–493.

Ziv E, Cauley J, Morin PA, Saiz R, Browner WS. Association between the T29→C polymorphism in the transforming growth factor β1 gene and breast cancer among elderly white women. The study of osteoporotic fractures. *JAMA.* 2001; 285:2859–2863.

Useful Web Resources

Biotechnology Resources

Agricultural biotechnology page. APHIS/USDA Web site. Available at: http://www.aphis.usda.gov/biotechnology/. Accessed December 29, 2001.

Agricultural biotechnology page. Department of Agriculture Web site. Available at: http://www.usda.gov/agencies/biotech/. Accessed July 31, 2002.

Agricultural Biotechnology Support Project. Michigan State University Web site. Available at: http://www.iia.msu.edu/absp/. Accessed July 31, 2002.

Annotated database of WWW sites pertaining to agricultural/environmental biotechnology. University of Vermont Web site. Available at: http://gophisb.biochem.vt.edu/othersites/indexlinksdblevel1.cfm. Accessed July 31, 2002.

Biotechnology: an information resource. National Agricultural Library page. Department of Agriculture Web site. Available at: http://www.nal.usda.gov/bic/. Accessed July 31, 2002.

Biotechnology page. FDA Center for Food Safety and Applied Nutrition (CFSAN) Web site. Available at: http://vm.cfsan.fda.gov/~lrd/biotechm.html. Accessed July 31, 2002.

Environmental Protection Agency Web site. Available at: http://www.epa.gov. Accessed July 31, 2002.

Featuring… agricultural biotechnology. ERS/USDA Web site. Available at: http://www.ers.usda.gov/Features/Biotech.htm. Accessed July 31, 2002.

Functional genomics: news, research, and resources on genomics and postgenomics. *Science* magazine Web site. Available at: http://www.sciencegenomics.org. Accessed July 31, 2002.

Genomes to Life: biological solutions for energy challenges. Department of Energy Web site. Available at: http://doegenomestolife.org/. Accessed July 31, 2002.

Information systems for biotechnology. University of Vermont Web site. Available at: http://www.isb.vt.edu/index.html. Accessed July 31, 2002.

Microarray project. NHGRI/NIH Web site. Available at: http://www.nhgri.nih.gov/DIR/Microarray/index.html. Accessed July 31, 2002.

OMIM: the Online Mendelian Inheritance of Man. National Center for Biotechnology Information/NIH Web site. Available at http://www3.ncbi.nlm.nih.gov/Omim. Accessed July 31, 2002.

U.S. regulatory oversight in biotechnology. APHIS/USDA Web site. Available at: www.aphis.usda.gov/biotech/OECD/usregs.htm. Accessed July 31, 2002.

5

Genetics and Medical Therapy

Except for the use of diagnostic testing over the past two decades, applications of genetic principles and genetic technologies to medicine have been limited. In the past, genetics was not recognized as central to medicine. Today genetics is seen as critical to preventive medicine and as heralding the era of personalized medicine.

As the molecular foundation for disease becomes known, it will be possible to prevent some of these diseases and to develop individualized approaches to others. Gene-based diagnostic testing will provide a tool for predicting individualized susceptibility to disease and response to therapy. Therapeutic options will include the development of bioengineered molecules such as human insulin and essential growth factors, gene therapy and stem cell therapy to correct faulty genes, stem cell therapy to regenerate tissues and organs damaged by disease, drugs prescribed to match an individual's genetic profile, and new drugs specifically bioengineered against vulnerable aspects of their targets. Medicine will be increasingly grounded in genetics.

This chapter will focus on genetic applications expected to have a major impact on the way medicine is practiced: diagnostic testing, therapeutic proteins, gene therapy, stem cell therapy, regenerative medicine, and pharmacogenomics.

GENETIC DIAGNOSTIC TESTING

Genetic testing is used to confirm the presence of a disorder and to provide information concerning the medical management of that disorder.

85

Individuals with a personal or family history of a particular disorder may use genetic testing as the basis for making personal decisions. Such testing is also useful for generating a molecular fingerprint of a person, animal, or microbe that can be used to establish identity or parentage of that organism. For infectious microorganisms, genetic testing also enables a clinical laboratory to quickly identify the organism and determine the antimicrobial agents to which it is susceptible.

What Types of Genetic Testing Are Available?

Genetic testing is performed for a wide variety of reasons. The major ones follow.

Diagnostic testing   Diagnostic testing is used to confirm or rule out a suspected disorder in an individual who demonstrates symptoms suggestive of that disorder. For example, the fasting blood sugar level is measured when diabetes is suspected, or catheterization may be performed when blockage of the coronary arteries is suspected. Diagnostic testing is commonly used in medicine today and is the type of testing with which we are more familiar. Testing the molecular composition of the DNA is a newer type of diagnostic test that can be used to determine whether an individual has the gene associated with a particular disease.

Predictive testing   Predictive testing is used for asymptomatic individuals with a family history of a particular disorder for which the specific gene mutation in that family can be identified. This type of testing can tell you whether you have the mutation but cannot tell you whether you will actually develop the disorder. Depending on the disorder, the particular mutation, and your lifestyle choices, you may have the gene and therefore the increased risk of developing the disorder that the mutation can cause, but you may not actually develop the disorder because of the influence of lifestyle choices on gene expression.

Predictive testing is medically indicated if early diagnosis enables the individual tested to make decisions that can reduce the risk of morbidity and mortality. In the absence of medical indications, predictive testing can provide the opportunity to make life-planning decisions. It can also eliminate the need for extra medical surveillance in those individuals found not to be at increased risk. For example, individuals at risk for colon cancer because of their family history undergo colonoscopy at regular intervals, sometimes annually. Individuals who have been found to be free of the gene that leads to colon cancer have the same risk of developing colon cancer as the general population and therefore no longer need to undergo frequent colonoscopies for medical surveillance purposes.

Both diagnostic and predictive testing can have profound psychosocial implications and should be accompanied by counseling from appropriate professionals. Those found to have a mutation that predisposes them to developing a disease are understandably anxious about their future and have a myriad of questions about what they can do to prevent the disease from developing. Family members who test negative for a disorder that runs in the family, particularly if debilitating, often have considerable survivor guilt, which psychosocial professionals can help alleviate.

At present, predictive testing of asymptomatic minors for adult-onset disorders is discouraged because of the strong psychosocial ramifications. For example, it is possible to test from birth for the presence of the gene that leads to midlife onset of the neurodegenerative Huntington's disease. There is considerable concern that those who know the child is at high risk (parents, family members, teachers, and others involved with nurturing the child's development) will possibly treat the child in a manner inconsistent with enabling that child to reach his or her full potential. The child is likely to experience considerable anxiety over his fate, particularly if the disorder has a one hundred percent chance of expression. For an in-depth treatment of the concerns about testing minors for disorders that will not develop until adulthood, see the policy statement by the American Society of Human Genetics/American College of Medical Genetics in the "Useful Resources" section of this chapter.

Carrier testing Carrier testing is for individuals who may be heterozygous (carriers) for a mutation inherited as a recessive trait, which means that the carrier individual would not be expected to have overt symptoms. Candidates for this type of testing include those with family members who have a disorder for which a genetic test is available, family members of a known carrier, and members of racial or ethnic groups known to have an elevated risk of developing a particular disorder. Usually the affected family member will also need to be tested in order to determine the particular mutation present in that family. This information then guides the specifics of the testing of the suspected carrier. Couples often request carrier testing when they are considering having a child and want to know whether they carry a genetic abnormality and what the chances will be that the child will inherit this abnormality.

Prenatal testing   Prenatal testing is carried out during a pregnancy to assess the health of the fetus when there is reason to believe the fetus is at risk for a disorder for which genetic testing is available. Common factors that increase risk include the age of the mother, genetic history of the mother, or her family history, race, or ethnicity. In the same way that testing minor children for adult-onset diseases is discouraged (see earlier section titled "Predictive testing"), prenatal testing for adult-onset disorders is controversial (see the policy statement by the American Society of Human Genetics/American College of Medical Genetics referenced in the "Useful Resources" section of this chapter for an in-depth exploration of the psychosocial issues).

Routine testing involves amniocentesis and/or chorionic villus sampling (CVS). More specialized testing includes placental biopsy, periumbilical blood sampling, and fetal skin biopsy via fetoscopy. Testing may be for chromosomal information or molecular genetics information, or both. Before molecular testing can be carried out, however, specific gene mutations must be identified in a carrier parent or an affected relative so that testing can assess the status of that particular DNA sequence in the fetus. Prenatal diagnostic testing carries some risk to both the fetus and the pregnancy.

Preimplantation testing   Preimplantation testing is an option when a couple is at high risk of producing a child with a serious medical condition. As an alternative to prenatal diagnosis and termination of an affected pregnancy, genetic analysis is performed on early embryos that result from in vitro fertilization. The availability of this service is limited at this time, but a successful use of this technique has been developed for early-onset Alzheimer's disease (Verlinsky et al., 2002). Costs are high and often not reimbursed by insurance. Because of the chance for error in preimplantation testing, the resulting pregnancies are often monitored by standard prenatal testing to be sure the fetus is free of the disease.

Newborn screening   Newborn screening is performed at birth and is intended to identify infants with an increased likelihood of developing specific disorders so that therapy can be started as soon as possible. Which disorders are screened varies from state to state. For those infants suspected of having a disorder, further diagnostic testing is indicated.

Identity testing Identity testing has a number of applications. Since each cell with a nucleus contains the full set of genetic material, any of a number of cell types can be used to develop a unique genetic fingerprint for an individual. Such DNA testing has been used in forensics for almost two decades. Parentage testing, particularly paternity testing, has also been a major application of DNA testing. Additionally, an infant can be DNA tested at birth, and this information serves as a unique identifier of that individual throughout life. Identifying victims of war, airplane and vehicle crashes, burns, murder, and other circumstances that change the human body beyond recognition has been made possible by using DNA-based testing. Among the famous mysteries in history that have been solved using genetic testing are the identification of the murdered Romanov family (the last czar of Russia, Nicholas II, his wife Alexandra, and their children) and of "the disappeared," children in Argentina in the 1970s whose grandparents had been searching for them.

Another type of identity testing involves detecting infectious organisms such as bacteria, fungi, and viruses in biological fluids or in food. The current methodology is slow and not as specific as DNA testing. Genetic testing requires only a probe that recognizes a DNA sequence unique to that organism, a more direct approach compared to current technology.

What's Involved in Genetic Testing?

Genetic testing provides a means of looking inside the individual to determine the genetic makeup, which is not obvious from just looking at the person or even testing him or her using standard medical diagnostic tests. Genetic testing can provide different levels of information about the genetic material, from the chromosomal level (called cytogenetic testing) to the DNA base level (called DNA-based testing). It can determine whether all the chromosomes are present and in their native forms–in other words, whether there are any major changes in the amount of genetic material or in its organizational structure. Testing can also determine the base sequence of a gene and detect whether there are any changes, compared with the normal sequence, that increase the risk of developing a health condition.

Genetic testing is already available for hundreds of genetic alterations and for the purpose of identifying an individual. A blood sample or cells from the inside of the cheek are typically used as the source of nucleated cells that contain the genetic material. However, all cells with nuclei contain genetic material, so it is also possible, and sometimes desirable, to use hair, skin, semen, or amniotic fluid as the starting material.

Cytogenetic Testing

Cytogenetic testing allows a picture (karyotype) to be constructed that accounts for each of the chromosomes and their partners. From this picture, it is possible to tell whether there is a change in the number of each chromosome. Earlier methodology involved staining the chromosomes. Each chromosome pair took on a characteristic banding pattern such that it was possible to determine whether any changes in the structure of a chromosome had occurred. More sophisticated and time-efficient methods of cytogenetic testing are now available, such as the FISH technique and spectral karyotyping (see Chapter 4, "Genetic Technologies," for details on chromosome visualization technology).

Karyotyping was the first type of genetic testing routinely available and was used to detect chromosomal abnormalities such as Down syndrome, in which an individual has three copies of all or a portion of chromosome 21. Karyotyping is used for amniocentesis and CVS when there is concern that the fetus may have a chromosomal abnormality. The typical cost of a cytogenetic test is between $500 and $600.

DNA-Based Genetic Testing

DNA-based genetic testing may be of several types. *Direct DNA testing* is used when a gene that causes a particular disorder has been identified and the changes in that gene can be detected and interpreted in terms of the impact on health. *Linkage testing* is used when the gene and its changes have not yet been identified. In this situation DNA regions coinherited with a disorder can be used as markers. The gene itself cannot be directly detected, but it is known that inheriting a particular marker is accompanied by the risk of also inheriting the disorder. The closer the marker is physically to the gene that causes the disorder, the higher the risk of inheriting the disorder each time the marker is inherited. The marker is typically unrelated to the disorder itself and is simply a convenient way to follow the inheritance of a gene when the actual base sequence of that gene is not yet known. A marker is essentially just another type of tag, much like the fluorescent probe. *Methylation testing* is used in disorders in which the degree to which the DNA is methylated influences disease development. Measuring the extent to which the DNA has attached methyl groups can be an indication of the risk of disease development. *Protein truncation testing* identifies mutations that result in a shortened protein product unable to perform its usual activities, which has detrimental effects on the function of the individual. The cost of DNA-based testing can range from $150 to $3,000, depending on the type of testing.

Who Performs Genetic Testing?

Genetic testing should be conducted only by qualified laboratories. In the United States, the Clinical Laboratory Improvement Act/Amendment of 1988 (CLIA) set standards for personnel qualifications, quality control systems, documentation, clinical testing procedures, and proficiency testing for clinical laboratories. On-site inspections of CLIA-approved labs are conducted every two years by regional or state agencies on behalf of the Centers for Medicare and Medicaid Services (CMS, formerly HCFA, the Health Care Financing Administration). Presently, there is no specialty certification for genetic testing, but the Clinical Laboratory Improvement Advisory Committee (CLIAC), the policy advisory body for CLIA, is considering legislation that will address the establishment of standardized requirements for genetic tests. At a minimum, laboratories should be approved by CLIA and have a history of performing the particular genetic test of interest. Most such laboratories at this time are located at large academic medical centers.

Which Labs Offer Genetic Testing?

To locate a laboratory that performs genetic testing for a particular disorder, visit the GeneTests Web site at http://www.genetests.org (GeneTests, Children's Hospital and Regional Medical Center, Seattle, WA 98105-0371). This site, funded by the National Library of Medicine of the NIH and the Maternal and Child Health Bureau of the Health and Rehabilitative Services Administration offers a searchable directory of medical laboratories that provide genetic testing as well as a directory that can be searched by disorder to find out whether a genetic test is available. For each disorder included, a list of laboratories that offer the genetic test for that disorder is provided. Through the GeneClinics portion of this program (funded by the NIH and developed at the University of Washington, Seattle), an expert-authored, peer-reviewed summary of the disorder is provided. The summary is updated regularly and includes the diagnosis, clinical description, differential diagnosis, management, genetic counseling, molecular genetics, references, and additional available resources for the disorder.

The Need for Informed Consent Prior to Genetic Testing

Many labs will not perform predictive testing unless the individuals to be tested have signed informed-consent forms and have received genetic counseling. Informed consent involves fully educating the individual about the following issues:

- The options for estimating risk that do not involve genetic testing
- The purpose of the testing
- The test procedure itself and its associated risks
- Sample collection specifics and logistics
- The technical accuracy of the test (sensitivity and specificity)
- Full disclosure of the fees associated with testing and counseling
- The information that will be generated by the testing and the fact that it may not be definitive
- The implications of either a positive or a negative result
- The options for therapeutic intervention
- The risk of the individual passing the mutation to children
- The possibility that other family members may need to be tested
- The psychological and social implications of the test results for individuals and their families
- The risk of insurance, employer, or social discrimination
- Confidentiality issues

Genetic Consultations

Depending on the particular health care professional conducting it, the genetics consultation can involve diagnosing, confirming, or ruling out a disorder; calculating and explaining the genetic risks; identifying and arranging for managing the various medical issues involved; and providing or arranging for psychosocial support.

The importance of accompanying genetic testing with psychosocial counseling cannot be overemphasized. People at risk for medical disorders have numerous questions and considerable emotional concerns. They need information on the disorder per se, what causes it, who else in the family could develop it, how that disorder could affect their health and well-being, and ways they can cope with the disorder. They need guidance as to whether they should be tested. If the test is positive and shows an increased risk of developing the disorder, these individuals often need psychosocial support for handling the outcome. If the test is negative, these individuals often experience guilt that they are unaffected when other family members are affected, and they too can benefit from psychosocial counseling. Since detection of a mutation does not guarantee that a disease will develop, people need assistance in sorting through what the test outcomes mean for their lives and the options available to them.

Fees for genetic consultations range from $50 to $300 and may or may not be reimbursed by third-party payers.

Qualified Genetics Professionals

There are a number of different types of genetics professionals. In the clinical setting, there may be a clinical geneticist (M.D., D.O., or Ph.D.), a genetic counselor (M.S.), or a nurse with a master's degree in genetics (M.S.N.). In the genetics testing laboratory, there will be a lab director (M.D., D.O., or Ph.D.) and possibly a genetic counselor. The M.D., D.O., and Ph.D. geneticists may opt for board certification through the American College of Medical Genetics.

THERAPEUTIC PROTEINS

Many diseases are caused by genetic mutations that result in an absent or dysfunctional protein. Being able to produce and deliver a functional version of the protein can mean the difference between life and death. A major technological hurdle that has to be overcome is where to get the normal protein in sufficient quantities. Proteins present in blood can be recovered and purified, but the process is expensive and carries the risk of contamination from infectious agents such as the viruses that cause acquired immunodeficiency syndrome (AIDS) and hepatitis. Other human tissues are not readily available for extraction. Not surprisingly, prior to the development of modern biotechnology, most therapeutic proteins, such as insulin for diabetes treatment, were obtained from slaughterhouse animals.

With the development of modern biotechnology methods, several alternative options became available for producing therapeutic proteins. Each had its own limitations but added an important step in advancing the production of therapeutic proteins on demand. For example, human cells can be grown in culture and made to express the protein of interest, which is then isolated and purified. This process is time-consuming, expensive, and only limited quantities are recovered. Microorganisms such as bacteria and yeast can be genetically engineered to express human proteins—in fact, bacteria were used to produce the first rDNA-derived human insulin. Proteins made by these microbes can be difficult to recover and often lack the modifications characteristic of mammalian proteins that are critical for activity in vivo. More recently, many of these hurdles have been overcome by the use of transgenic animals that secrete the therapeutic proteins in their milk, such as sheep, goats, and cattle. Output is high, cost is low, and the proteins are fully processed with the appropriate modifications. The therapeutic protein alpha$_1$ antitrypsin for treating cystic fibrosis is now in clinical trial.

Recombinant DNA–Derived Proteins

There are two major types of therapeutic proteins: those derived from recombinant DNA and those derived from monoclonal antibodies. To develop a therapeutic protein using rDNA technology, the gene that codes for the therapeutic protein must be identified first. Thanks to restriction enzyme technology, that gene can then be cut from the DNA of human cells and pasted into a production vector, which may be a bacterium, a plant, or perhaps cells from the mammary glands of a goat or cow. If engineered properly, expression of the transplanted gene can be switched on, and the protein is synthesized. The protein must then be recovered and purified from the production medium. Examples of recombinant proteins used therapeutically include insulin for diabetes, tissue plasminogen activator (tPA) for dissolving blood clots during the early stages of a heart attack or stroke, beta-type naturietic peptide (hBNP) for the short-term management of congestive heart failure, the hormone erythropoietin for stimulation of red blood cell production and helping against the anemia that accompanies chronic renal failure, the human growth hormone for hypophyseal dwarfism, a vaccine against hepatitis B infection, and various cellular messaging molecules such as the interferons and interleukins.

Monoclonal Antibody–Derived Proteins

Monoclonal antibody–derived proteins are another promising therapeutic approach but involve quite a different mechanism. Antibodies are produced by immune cells in response to the detection of foreign proteins in the body. Each antibody recognizes and binds to a specific, minute region of the protein. Ultimately that single antibody-producing cell grows into a colony of cells, all producing the single, highly specific antibody protein called a monoclonal antibody. Biotechnology advances have allowed the fusion of monoclonal antibody–producing cells with cells that divide continuously, thereby creating cellular factories for the production of a particular monoclonal antibody, itself a therapeutic protein. Monoclonals, as they are called, were an early outcome of biotechnology applied to medicine, but they have only recently begun to live up to their therapeutic promise (see Chapter 4, "Genetic Technologies," for more details on the discussion of monoclonal antibody technology).

A major expected application of monoclonals involves the antibody's ability to specifically identify and bind to a cell surface protein (antigen) unique to a cancer cell. The attached monoclonal can be exploited in three ways: to tag the cancer cells so they can be located, to deliver a toxic drug to the cancer cells but not to normal cells, or to target the cancer cell for destruction because, once the binding occurs, the immune response is then set in motion and ultimately results in killing the cell to which the antibody is attached. Monoclonals used successfully in the clinic include rituximab (Rituxan, Genetech, Inc., South San Francisco, Calif.) for non-Hodgkin's lymphoma and trastuzumab (Herceptin, Genetech, Inc., South San Francisco, Calif.) for breast cancer. Rituximab works by binding to an antigen expressed on the surface of the cancer cell. It is not the ideal monoclonal in that the antigen it targets, CD20, is also expressed on normal B lymphocytes (immune cells). Rituximab does, however, produce partial or total remission in many patients, and the normal immune cells appear to recover without permanent damage.

Trastuzumab is another clinically useful monoclonal antibody but works by a mechanism different from that of rituximab. Trastuzumab is used for patients with metastatic breast cancer who are considered to have a poor prognosis. These cancers frequently overexpress the protein HER-2. This application again makes use of monoclonals' ability to bind to protein targets, in this case the HER-2 receptor, but centers on their ability to interfere with key intracellular communication activities. Many of the messaging molecules responsible for communication within and between cells work by binding to protein receptors and triggering a cascade of events (often involving tyrosine kinase) that then sends a signal to the interior of the receiving cell. The HER-2 protein is a tyrosine kinase receptor involved in signal transduction. If the HER-2 receptor is already occupied by a monoclonal antibody, the signal cannot bind, which disrupts the intracellular signal transduction process. Alternatively, if the signaling molecule were a protein, a monoclonal could be developed that would be able to bind to the signal itself, preventing both its binding to the receptor and activation of the communication cascade.

When the disrupted process is an inflammatory cascade, monoclonal antibody interference is a desirable action. Several examples of these types of applications exist. The drug infliximab (Remicade, Centocor, Inc., Malvern, Pa.) is an anti-inflammatory agent used for inflammatory bowel disorders. It prevents the proinflammatory cytokine tumor necrosis factor alpha (TNF-α) from binding to its cell surface receptors. Etanercept (Enbrel, Amgen, Inc., Thousand Oaks, Calif.), used for rheumatoid arthritis, similarly ties up cytokines and prevents them from binding to their receptors and initiating the inflammatory cascade.

A number of therapeutic proteins and monoclonal antibodies have been approved by the U.S. Food and Drug Administration (FDA), and many more are in clinical trials.

GENE THERAPY

Gene therapy involves adding genes to cells to change the way those cells work or, potentially, modifying gene expression such that a gene's protein product is not expressed. The goal can be to treat or cure an existing disease or to prevent the development of a disease. Gene therapy can involve somatic or germ-line cells. With somatic gene therapy, the change will affect individuals for their lifetimes but will not be passed along to their offspring. With germ-line gene therapy, the parents' egg and sperm cells are altered, and the changes then pass to the offspring.

Obviously gene therapy represents a powerful technology with the potential for treating disease by correcting the underlying faulty genes, but it also has the potential for misuse. The technology is still quite young. Much remains to be worked out in terms of technical details and ethical, legal, and social implications. Several experimental applications for somatic gene therapy have been tried since 1990, and many more are currently in progress. Germ-line gene therapy in human beings is not conducted at this time because of ethical and safety concerns (Frankel and Chapman, 2000), but it has been successfully accomplished in other primates. Preimplantation testing is sometimes confused with germ-line gene therapy. In preimplantation testing, a fertilized egg that is tested to be free of the disease gene of concern is selected for implantation. In this case genetic information is being used for selection; no change in the genetic material takes place. In gene therapy, by contrast, the egg (or sperm) is engineered so that the defective gene is corrected prior to fertilization and implantation.

Hurdles in the Development of Gene Therapy

In addition to the ethical concerns, there are technological hurdles facing gene therapy before it can become commonplace. A major hurdle is the need for vectors, delivery vehicles that shuttle the gene into the body. Like an astronaut in a space capsule, the gene has to be transported in a vehicle that can protect it from the unfriendly external environment while maintaining favorable conditions inside the capsule. When the capsule arrives at the target, there must be a way to transport the astronaut (the gene) safely from the interior of the capsule into the new environment in order to function properly.

The most common vectors presently are viruses. Viruses actually have the type of structure described above: a protective outer capsule and a means of injecting their inner core of genetic material into human cells. By inserting the beneficial human gene into the viral genome, scientists have had some success in introducing genes into human beings. The virus delivery system is not, however, without its drawbacks—toxic reactions, immune responses, inflammation, problems with controlling gene expression, and missing the target. Alternative approaches to a viral delivery system are physical mechanisms such as injecting the DNA into the cells (microinjection), using electrical current to make the cell membrane porous so that DNA can move into the cell (electroporation), and using vehicles that enclose the genetic material in a bubble of fat (a structure called a liposome) so that the delivery system can fuse with the human cell membrane and bring the gene into the cell. Once inside, the gene must be transported to the nucleus and expressed. In some instances the gene integrates itself into the host's genetic material; in others the gene remains physically separate from the host's DNA but is still expressed.

A second major hurdle is our still-primitive understanding of the basic science of gene expression. One of the first steps in such therapy is to locate the tissue(s) in which the gene is active. Although every nucleated cell contains the full genetic information, every tissue does not express every gene. It's important, then, to get the therapeutic gene into the tissue that requires it and into a sufficient number of cells in that tissue. Initially the focus will be on those diseases that primarily affect a single tissue. Tissue-targeted vectors would be more likely to transfer the gene into a sufficient number of cells so that the tissue can function normally. The LDL-C receptor involves liver cells and represents a useful target for gene therapy. However, type 2 diabetes involves multiple tissues and will be a more difficult gene therapy to develop.

Even after the gene is successfully delivered to the target tissue by the vector, it does not always find a warm welcome. Cells have so-called gene silencing mechanisms, whereby they can turn off the expression of the therapeutic gene. Methylation is one such mechanism that is a fundamental strategy cells normally use to prevent specific regions of DNA from being expressed. By attaching methyl groups to the therapeutic gene, cells can prevent its expression and its therapeutic effects. In time, advances in genetic engineering should be able to circumvent these difficulties.

Our understanding of the function of most human genes is still quite primitive. Without having the big picture readily available, it is quite possible that a single gene may have more than one function or that correcting one problem will precipitate another, unexpected one. For example, sometimes carriers of a genetic disorder have a survival advantage over those who have two normal copies of the gene. An example is sickle cell disease. Having two copies of the gene that codes for sickle cell hemoglobin produces a deadly condition. However, red blood cells of individuals with one gene for sickle cell hemoglobin and one for normal hemoglobin are hostile environments for the malaria parasite and thereby provide a survival advantage to such carrier individuals compared with those who have two copies of the gene coding for normal hemoglobin.

As with any new technology, a major hurdle is changing from the small-scale production methods used in the research laboratory to the large-scale production necessary for commercial application. This conversion process always seems fraught with challenges, and gene therapy is no exception. Using live cells as vectors is accompanied by many uncertainties. The cells are at risk of contamination from viruses, and the vector cells contain their own genetic material and expression apparatus that are not readily controlled and may introduce complications into the process.

Financial hurdles are proving as challenging as the technological hurdles. The original promise of gene therapy was thought to be the treatment of diseases for which there are no cures, disorders such as sickle cell disease, cystic fibrosis, Huntington's disease, and severe combined immunodeficiency disease. Such disorders are ideal for gene therapy because they typically involve the alteration of a single gene. Inserting a functional copy of the gene would be a logical approach to correcting the inherited dysfunction. The hurdle is that the research and clinical trials required to develop such therapy are expensive, and because the number of individuals with these disorders is small, the market is limited. Significant investment on the part of pharmaceutical or biotechnology companies is necessary to develop such therapies, but the market provides little financial incentive for them.

Instead, the focus has shifted to diseases with large markets, such as cancer and AIDS. Unlike the single-gene disorders, these common diseases are more complex and more difficult to address with gene therapy at this time; thus progress is expected to be slow.

Specific Applications of Gene Therapy

Given the formidable hurdles that gene therapy has had to overcome, it's not surprising that few successes exist at this early stage. One of the first reports of success concerns using gene therapy to treat familial hypercholesterolemia (FH), in which the LDL-C receptors in the liver are defective (Grossman et al., 1994). Cholesterol cannot enter the liver to be degraded, so it is left to circulate in the bloodstream and ultimately to accumulate in the blood vessels and produce severe atherosclerosis. In this disorder, the target cells are liver cells. Liver tissue is removed from the individual with FH, and the cells are separated and grown (cultured) in the laboratory. In the culture medium is a viral vector containing the healthy FH gene that codes for a functional liver cholesterol receptor. The cultured cells now infected with the virus are returned to the liver of the individual with FH through the portal vein. As the new liver cells begin to produce functional LDL-C receptors, the individual's cholesterol levels drop.

Another success of gene therapy has been with severe combined immunodeficiency disease (SCID), a disease made famous in the early 1980s by a young boy named David, known worldwide as "the boy in the bubble." The immune system is completely crippled by SCID (pronounced "skid"); children born with this disease are extremely susceptible to infections and have had to live inside a germ-free, airtight chamber resembling a bubble in order to survive. Multiple defective genes give rise to SCID; again, understanding the basic science underlying each disease is critical to successful gene therapy. Gene therapy for certain types of the disease is now available, in which infants are treated by introducing healthy genes into their immune cells so that they have functional immune systems (Cavazzana-Calvo et al., 2000).

The type of gene therapy used for treating FH and SCID is called ex vivo gene therapy, meaning the genetic transfer takes place *outside* the body. Cells are removed from the individuals and grown in culture, the normal gene is introduced into the cells, and the cells are then returned to the individuals. In contrast, in vivo gene therapy is used when the cells that express the disorder are not readily removed and the faulty gene needs to be corrected *inside* the body.

Cystic fibrosis (CF) is a good example of the need for in vivo gene therapy. Unfortunately, successful gene therapy for this disease has been elusive. The mutation that causes it disables the cystic fibrosis transmembrane conductance regulator (*CFTR*) gene, which leads to defects in ion transport across the membranes of lung cells and in other mucous membranes of the body. Thick mucus builds up in the lungs and pancreas so that digestive enzymes cannot be secreted normally. Normal lung function is disrupted, and the thick mucus sets the stage for recurring infection. Gene therapy has targeted the cells that line the lungs and has focused on finding a vector that normally attacks the lung cells and injects its DNA, such as the common cold virus, that would carry the healthy CF gene and inject it into lung cells. Unfortunately, success has been hampered by the limitations of the delivery vector, and new vectors are being investigated. The basic premise for the gene therapy approach to this disease is sound; however, technical hurdles still need to be surmounted.

For more complex disorders such as cancer and AIDS, other approaches are used. Thus far the AIDS virus has outsmarted every attempt to eliminate or even control it. For cancer, though, the picture is more encouraging. Two different strategies are under investigation. One is oriented toward enhancing the body's defense against the cancer cells or at least protecting the body's innate defense system against present treatments for eradicating cancer, such as chemotherapy. The other strategy focuses on killing only the cancer cells. For example, in chemotherapy the drugs used to kill the cancer cells also wreak havoc on the body's immune cells. A gene that confers multiple drug resistance could be introduced into immune cells so that the cancer cells would die and the individual's immune cells would survive. Another approach is to target tumor cells and invade them with a virus that carries a so-called suicide gene. Expression of the gene leads to the destruction of the cell in which it is expressed. To date neither approach has produced resounding success. Again, the theoretical bases are sound; the technical difficulties remain to be overcome.

Gene therapy or clinical trials are in progress for a number of human diseases:

- Inborn errors of metabolism disorders: galactosemia, Gaucher's disease, Fanconi's anemia, Hunter's syndrome, and urea cycle disorders

- Blood disorders such as sickle cell disease, beta thalassemia, and hemophilia B
- Cardiovascular disease such as flow-limiting coronary artery and peripheral vascular disease, hypertension, and hypercholesterolemia
- Muscle disorders such as the muscular dystrophies
- Rheumatoid arthritis
- Neurological disorders such as Alzheimer's disease
- A number of lung diseases: cystic fibrosis, alpha$_1$ antitrypsin deficiency, pulmonary inflammation, surfactant deficiency, lung cancer, malignant mesothelioma, and pulmonary hypertension
- Numerous cancer types besides lung cancer: breast cancer, colon cancer, glioblastoma and other brain tumors, melanoma, non-Hodgkin's lymphoma, ovarian cancer, pancreatic cancer, and bladder cancer

In spite of the hurdles, which are not unusual for any new technology as it finds its way to large-scale application, somatic gene therapy looks quite promising. Clearly, successful application requires not only technological tools and know-how but also fundamental understanding of the disease, the gene(s) involved, and the cells primarily affected by the dysfunctional gene(s). This type of basic research and insight into the details of the human body and what constitutes wellness and illness is a major focus of the Human Genome Project and is expected to contribute significantly to the advancement of gene therapy as a disease treatment option.

ELSI-Related Concerns

There are many ethical, legal, and social issues (ELSI) connected with gene therapy. What exactly is normal? How is a disease or disorder defined, as compared with a disability? Do disabilities need to be cured or prevented? How will society handle the capability of permanently curing a disease, as opposed to treating it in the presenting individual for his or her lifetime only? If gene therapy remains expensive, who will have access to it? Who will pay for it? If there are affordable gene therapies that will cure or at least lessen a disease or disability, will society expect everyone to take advantage of them? If someone does not and goes on to develop a lifelong medical limitation, should the individual be expected to bear the expense of that limitation, or should society? What about individuals who have a rare single-gene disorder for which there is little financial incentive to develop gene therapies? Should such individuals be denied the medical care they need? How do we as a society balance the needs of a company to make a reasonable profit and the needs of society to provide for the most limited of its members?

The tragic death of an 18-year-old patient in a gene therapy trial in 1999 and the discovery of a death at another medical center that was not properly reported heightened concern about the safety of gene therapy trials. As a result, the NIH and the FDA have moved to increase oversight of such trials. The Gene Therapy Clinical Trial Monitoring Plan was established to improve protection of participants in gene therapy trials. The Gene Transfer Safety Symposia initiative was developed to educate researchers and participants about safety, good clinical practice in research, entry criteria for gene therapy trials, the importance of informed consent, and other key issues relevant to such trials.

STEM CELL THERAPY AND REGENERATIVE MEDICINE

An alternative to germ-line gene therapy is cell therapy using either fetal or stem cells. The fertilized egg at its beginning has a full complement of genetic information and is capable of dividing and differentiating into the wide variety of cell types that will form the adult organs and ultimately a complete organism. Embryonic (or fetal) cells can be grown in the laboratory, be differentiated into a variety of tissue types, and serve as the starting point for treating individuals with a variety of diseases that require tissue repair or regeneration. There are, however, many ELSI-related concerns surrounding the use of fetal tissue that may limit its applications. Fetal tissue research has been conducted on an experimental basis with promising results, particularly for neurological diseases such as Parkinson's and Alzheimer's diseases. However, a recent, carefully controlled study in which cells from aborted fetuses were implanted into individuals with Parkinson's disease was disappointing (Freed et al., 2001). Although participants sixty years old or younger improved with the transplant, it worked too well in approximately fifteen percent of the participants, and the excess neurotransmitter that was produced led to involuntary jerking and writhing movements. The outcome of this trial has rekindled a heated debate over whether the use of fetal cells for human research is appropriate. Many predict that the future of research using fetal tissue has been seriously jeopardized by the findings in this study.

Fortunately, there is an alternative in the use of stem cells rather than fetal cells for gene therapy. Stem cells are undifferentiated cells. Because they contain the full set of genetic information, the potential exists for these cells to become whichever type of differentiated cell is desired. In a developing organism, the vast majority of cells within a tissue normally move past the stem cell stage and differentiate into the highly specialized cell type characteristic of that tissue: cardiac muscle, liver, bone marrow, and so on. Within these cell populations, however, are also undifferentiated stem cells. Some tissues such as the bone marrow, skin, and small intestine maintain a pool of stem cells that can be used to generate new tissue as needed. In fact, the stem cells from bone marrow form the basis for bone marrow transplantation for individuals with malignancies and other diseases of blood cells. It has long been thought, however, that other organs such as the brain, heart, and kidneys as well as the nervous system did not contain stem cells and that, once differentiated, cells from these tissues could not be reprogrammed to return to their beginnings and differentiate into new types of cells.

Recent developments suggest much more is possible in this area than originally thought. Stem cells have been found in organs such as the brain and muscle. Both cell culture and animal studies suggest that these cells can be grown in the laboratory; implanted into brain or muscle tissue; differentiated into mature, specialized cells; and function appropriately for their tissue type. Furthermore, stem cells isolated from one tissue can be made to differentiate into a variety of unrelated cell types. These successes open the door to regenerating organs using an individual's own stem cells (regenerative medicine) and potentially to cloning whole organisms.

For medical purposes, the fact that bone marrow stem cells have been made to differentiate into skeletal muscle cells, liver cells, or nerve cells raises the possibility of using these cells to treat disorders such as the muscular dystrophies and Parkinson's disease, liver disorders, and stroke. It may be possible to take stem cells from the individual to be treated and differentiate them into the desired type of cell needed for implantation. Similarly, stem cells could be made to develop into hearts, livers, and other organs currently in short supply for transplantation. Using stem cells from the individual needing the transplant would circumvent the immune response and rejection risk that accompanies transplantation as well as the need for lifelong immunosuppressive drugs.

PHARMACOGENOMICS

Pharmacogenomics is the application of genetic technology to drug therapy and is expected to be an early practical outcome of the Human

Genome Project. In spite of the life-saving benefits that medications bring to millions of people, their use is not without significant risk. Drugs that are effective for one person with asthma or depression or high blood pressure are ineffective for another and may even cause serious side effects. Similar situations can be found with virtually all drugs. Although many factors affect drug efficacy and toxicity, the one thought to have the greatest influence is an individual's genetic makeup.

Genetic variation among individuals influences not only the metabolism and disposition of drugs by altering the enzymes responsible for drug conversions in the body but also the targets, such as membrane receptors, that drugs bind to in order to exert their effects. These individual differences have been known since the 1950s. Until recently, however, the tools for identifying these inherited differences were not available. Now it's possible to pinpoint how individuals differ genetically and to associate specific genetic differences with particular drug responses. Initially, pharmacogenomics is expected to focus on two areas: drug response genotyping and targeted drug development.

Drug response genotyping involves using a person's genetic information to predict whether a particular drug will be beneficial or harmful to that person. Prescribing drugs based on an individual's metabolic profile would be preferable to the current practice of prescribing based on a so-called average response. Clinicians are aware that the one-size-fits-all approach is inappropriate, but until the present advances in genomic research, individualization has not been possible. By using gene-based diagnostic tests to generate genetic profiles of individuals, however, it will be possible to divide patients into those who are likely to respond positively to a particular drug (responders) and those who will not (nonresponders). The ability to pinpoint the subgroups that will be most helped or harmed by particular medications promises improved patient care and more effective utilization of resources. The physician will be able to select drugs that best match the patient's likelihood of benefiting from them and to avoid giving a drug to a patient who is genetically predisposed to having a toxic reaction to it.

Targeted drug development involves identifying points at which a physiological process can be interrupted and making a drug whose action disrupts this process. These research efforts can improve drug efficacy and decrease the incidence of adverse side effects. Enzymes and receptor-ligand pairs have historically been the main targets of drugs, but any step critical to the survival of a cell, tumor, or organism is a potential target for drug intervention.

Together these two approaches, which acknowledge and work with differences in individual genetic makeup, will help physicians match the right drug to the right person in the right dosage to get the job done without unwanted side effects. They also hold the promise of decreasing the cost of health care by decreasing the cost of bringing new drugs to market. Newer technology promises a shortening of the drug development process at considerable savings. Clinical trials are extremely costly in terms of both time and expense, yet the vast majority of drugs never make it through clinical testing and onto the market because of problems with efficacy or safety. These problems are now recognized as owing to genetic heterogeneity. An additional cost-effective step being considered is to retest those drugs that have previously failed clinical trials once the basic molecular biology is known. These drugs may be just right for certain subpopulations or even for the majority, once the population that responds negatively is eliminated from consideration for treatment with these drugs.

Drug Response Genotyping

Variability in drug response among individuals results from individual variation in the DNA sequence within drug-metabolizing genes. The key enzymes are the CYP450s, of which multiple distinct enzymes have been characterized in human beings, and *N*-acetyltransferase (NAT2). The genes coding for these enzymes are known to occur in multiple alleles, and many are polymorphic. Many of these variants affect the function of the enzyme product. Just how function is affected in each enzyme variant depends on the specific mutation and can result in the final enzyme being unaffected or having greater or lesser activity than its supposedly normal counterpart.

Interestingly, polymorphisms have been described for most of the drug-metabolizing enzymes, and the degree of polymorphism (how many variants exist per gene) appears to be high. These enzymes are critical to a drug's effectiveness and safety. The physician presently sets the drug dosage based on weight and the assumption that the patient has drug-metabolizing activity typical of the average person. Benefiting from the drug depends on that enzymatic machinery being able to metabolize the drug to a form that is both active (to do the job intended) and soluble (so that the metabolized drug can ultimately be excreted from the body). Unmetabolized drug is almost always toxic; the goal, then, is to give an individual just enough drug so that he or she can metabolize it fully and generate the concentration level necessary to take care of the problem being addressed. An individual with a mutation that decreases the function of the enzyme that metabolizes a particular drug will not reach the therapeutic level within the expected time; therefore the drug will be less effective for this individual. There will also be more unmetabolized drug in his or her body than anticipated, so the drug will be less safe for such an individual. Individuals with mutations that result in metabolizing the drug faster than the norm will clear that drug more rapidly. No toxic residues should remain, which is positive, but these individuals may achieve a higher-than-expected concentration of drug in their systems faster than expected, which may be harmful, and the drug will not be available for the full length of time needed. Such individuals are typically characterized as resistant to therapy with particular drugs. In the middle are the majority of people with two normal alleles, with one normal and one mutant, or with two mutant alleles that have minimal impact on function.

Examples of the effects of polymorphism in drug-metabolizing enzymes are commonplace in medicine. The NAT2 enzyme is responsible for metabolizing a variety of arylamine and hydrazine drugs as well as several carcinogens. Numerous mutations that result in decreased function of this enzyme have been described and, not surprisingly, numerous drug toxicity effects have been described for individuals with polymorphisms that result in slow acetylation. Examples include isoniazid-induced neurotoxicity, hydrazine-induced lupus, dye-associated bladder cancer, and sulfonamide-induced hypersensitivity reactions.

Polymorphism in the CYP450 genes has similar consequences. Changes in the CYP2D6 enzyme alone affects the metabolism of over forty drugs. Both slow metabolizers and ultrarapid metabolizers have been reported. Researchers investigating the association between polymorphisms in the CYP2C9 enzyme and the safety and efficacy of the anticoagulation drug warfarin found that certain polymorphisms are associated with an increased risk of overanticoagulation and increased risk of bleeding (Higashi et al., 2002). What's mind-boggling here is that there are multiple distinct CYP450 enzymes, each with a number of variants. Obviously the individual variation is extensive, with far-reaching physiological consequences, not just for drugs but for all the potentially toxic molecules that the CYP450 systems of the digestive tract and liver must biotransform to less toxic, more soluble compounds that can be eliminated from the body.

Beyond the drug-metabolizing enzymes themselves, the ability to pinpoint other genes an individual carries can be helpful in matching drugs and genotypes. For example, having the *APOE* genotype that has been associated with late-onset Alzheimer's disease appears to predict who will respond poorly to the drug tacrine, a cholinesterase inhibitor used to increase the low levels of acetylcholine that characterize Alzheimer's disease (Farlow et al., 1996). Those with the *APOE4* genotype (*E4/E4* homozygotes) respond poorly to tacrine when compared to individuals with other alleles at this gene locus. Furthermore, a drug may appear not to work for a population as a whole but, when classified by genotypes, may be beneficial for particular groups. In a clinical trial of an experimental drug for Alzheimer's that involved four hundred subjects, the results for the population as a whole were disappointing. However, when the researchers classified the population by *APOE* genotype, those subjects with the *E4/E4* genotype were actually helped by the drug.

Another important factor in determining efficacy and side effects is the genetic influence on the ability of a drug to interact with its target. For example, genetic changes can result in changes in the structure of receptors on the cell surface that either enhance or diminish a drug's ability to bind. An interesting example of this situation is with individuals with schizophrenia who do not respond to the usual psychotropic drugs. Many in this subpopulation respond to the antipsychotic drug clozapine, which binds to receptors for a number of neurotransmitters, including serotonin. The ability of these individuals to respond to clozapine is believed to result from polymorphisms in their serotonin receptors (Arranz et al., 1998).

Another example linking genetic makeup and drug-metabolizing ability has been reported for the asthma drug albuterol, which targets the beta$_2$ adrenergic receptors of lung tissue. When activated, these receptors cause the smooth muscle tissues of the lung to relax, which results in dilation of the bronchioles and opening of the airways. The gene for this receptor is polymorphic. Researchers identified twelve patterns of SNPs that directly affect response to the medication, making it possible to identify asthma sufferers who will respond well to the drug and those who will not (Drysdale et al., 2000).

When one considers that every individual is an amalgam of polymorphisms representing each of the drug-metabolizing enzymes and that many people use multiple medications, it becomes obvious that prescribing pharmaceuticals is a complicated and risky process. Luckily, extensive data are available concerning which enzymes metabolize which drugs. What is needed now is a way to identify genetic differences in individuals and correlate them with functional enzyme activity. Such studies are called *association studies* and can directly correlate a particular level of function of each drug-metabolizing enzyme with a specific gene. It then becomes possible to develop a diagnostic test in which it can be determined which variant of each enzyme a patient has, thereby giving the physician the ability to predict how that patient will metabolize each drug. Such tests will be based on the ability to identify SNPs, as discussed in detail in Chapter 4.

Basing drug decisions on genetic makeup is logical. The technology is progressing such that using genetic variation to predict drug response should be feasible in the near future. Expect the initial progress to focus on single-gene effects on drug metabolism and to move, in time, to an even more complex situation, where drug response is an effect of multiple genes and their interactions with environmental factors.

However, classifying patients according to their genetic profile, even for the beneficial purposes of maximizing positive drug response and minimizing toxic responses, is of concern to many. There are numerous drug-metabolizing differences among the various racial and ethnic groups. Could drug response profiling lead to further divisions among the races?

Furthermore, from an economic standpoint, individualizing pharmaceuticals may also be an unpopular strategy with drug companies. Their orientation historically has been to seek blockbuster drugs that will return a substantial profit and offset the multimillion-dollar development costs for those drugs. If drugs had to be tailored to specific subpopulations, several drugs might be needed for a single condition. The market for each drug is likely to be significantly less than for a single drug, thereby diminishing the economic return for the company.

Targeted Drug Development

Drug development involves identifying a biological target whose function can be modified, typically by an organic molecule of small molecular weight, a peptide or protein, or a monoclonal antibody. Sample targets are the enzymes and factors involved with duplicating and expressing the genetic information; receptors and molecules in cell surface membranes; protein kinases, phosphatases, and proteases involved in intracellular communication; hormones, growth factors, cytokines, and neurotransmitters involved in communication between cells; and any component unique to a tumor or infectious organism. Targeting a drug's action is expected to minimize the magnitude of undesirable side effects and increase the effectiveness of the drug.

Genetic research is expected to result in many enhancements to the drug development process. The following include some of the more promising:

- **An increased number of potential targets for drug intervention.** It is estimated that only about five hundred of the potential five thousand different targets in the human body are currently used for drug design. Genomics research is expected to significantly expand the identification of potential targets by broadening the understanding of basic physiological processes and the sequence of events linking genes with disease.

- **Generation of new targets for antimicrobial drugs that do not overlap with human targets.** The Human Genome Project includes the sequencing of the genomes of a number of microorganisms. Using the sophisticated computer technology being developed, the genomes of these organisms can be searched for sequences common to the infectious microbes but absent in human beings. Proteins encoded by these sequences are potential targets for drug intervention, presumably with minimal side effects.

- **A supply of new tools for validating drug targets.** As the genomes of numerous model organisms commonly used for research purposes are sequenced and the encoded proteins and their functions are deciphered, these organisms will become tools for testing whether a new drug hits its target in the manner hypothesized at the time of drug design. Species seemingly unrelated to human beings, such as the fruit fly or roundworm, are useful models because they share many of the same genes and physiological processes of more complex organisms such as human beings.

- **Development of improved vaccines.** Genomic research will give rise to vaccines containing DNA and RNA from several pathogens. The genetic material in these vaccines will give rise to antigens able to stimulate an immune response but unable to cause infection, two qualities that current vaccines have been unable to combine.

- **A potential reduction in drug development costs.** Presently the path from design to market availability of a drug is lengthy and expensive. Many experimental, animal, and clinical trials are required to ensure safety of the final product. Even with this laborious process, the number of adverse reactions from properly prescribed drugs is high (Lazarou et al., 1998). With improved drug design and better validation of new drugs prior to clinical trials, it will be possible to eliminate inappropriate drugs early in the process so that only those drugs with a low risk-to-benefit ratio will make it to the clinical trial stage, which should greatly decrease the number of clinical trial failures. These fundamental improvements in the process of bringing a new drug to market should save considerable time and money and will hopefully be reflected in the market price of the drug.

■ **Minimization of hepatotoxicity.** Liver toxicity is an ongoing concern with drugs and is often not detected until the clinical trial stage or even after a drug is on the market, as was the experience with troglitazone, an oral antihyperglycemic agent used to improve insulin sensitivity in individuals with type 2 diabetes. Understanding the molecular mechanisms of hepatotoxicity and identification of the critical susceptibility genes and molecular targets is expected to result in screening tools that will predict which drugs are most likely to cause liver toxicity and which individuals will be most susceptible to such damage.

Clearly, DNA sequence information alone cannot provide all the answers drug companies need. Additional aspects of genetic research will be needed to support the development of pharmacogenomics, specifically functional genomics, which involves identifying the role of gene protein products, and bioinformatics (computational genomics), which provides the tools for organizing, storing, retrieving, and using in a meaningful way the massive database of information generated.

IMPLICATIONS FOR THE NUTRITION PROFESSIONAL

As a member of the medical team, the nutrition professional will need to be familiar with the changes genetics is bringing to medical therapy. Ultimately we will know enough about an individual's genotype to be able to predict the diseases for which he or she is at greatest risk and to develop therapies with the goal of preventing the manifestation of those disorders. Physicians will be able to predict how an individual will react to environmental stresses and to particular medical therapies. The individual referred to a nutrition professional will come with new types of test results, drug prescriptions, medical therapies, and ultimately a prescription requesting the development of a nutrition plan that addresses his or her particular genotype. He or she will have stem cell–regenerated organ transplants. There will be far more interest in genetic family history and its impact on the individual's health potential. At the very least, people will expect the nutrition professional to be conversant about these various aspects of their treatment. At most, the nutrition professional will be expected to analyze the genetic information, to convert it into targeted nutrition therapies, and to help people sort out the complex scientific and psychosocial aspects of their care.

Genetic testing will likely become commonplace. As the Human Genome Project identifies genes and links them with susceptibility to disease, the number of tests will increase. Nutrition professionals will be expected to provide nutrition therapy for the particular disorders identified and will need to continuously update knowledge, both their own and that of their clients. Nutrition professionals will also be called upon to provide psychosocial support to the client and his or her family members.

Gene therapy is a powerful technological tool that presents many soul-searching questions for society. The debate has just begun. As citizens, each of us should weigh in with considered opinions on these issues. As nutrition professionals, we will be faced with developing therapies to complement the new genetic makeup of clients. It will be important to understand technological developments and their functional implications for the client. The extent to which the client's function has been restored will be an important factor in developing nutrition therapies.

Regarding pharmacogenomics, as nutrition professionals we are concerned about the potential for drug interactions with foods clients eat or dietary supplements they may be taking. Research is beginning to provide a clearer picture of how drugs work mechanically, which helps us to predict potential interactions. The technology applied to drug-related enzymes and receptors will also be applied to food digestion and absorption. Nutrition practice may well focus considerably more on matching foods to an individual's genetically determined food-processing machinery.

Pharmacogenomics is of interest to us as citizens because it promises us drugs that are more effective, safer, and possibly less expensive. It will become commonplace for the primary care physician to perform a quick genotyping on a sample of cells from a cheek swab and then prescribe medications that match our individualized profiles with regard to drug-metabolizing capability. This advancement alone should greatly decrease the possibility of adverse reactions from drug therapy.

Useful Resources

American Society of Human Genetics/American College of Medical Genetics. ASHG/ACMG report. Points to consider: ethical, legal, and psychosocial implications of genetic testing in children and adolescents. *Am J Hum Genet.* 1995; 57:1233–1241.

Arranz MJ, Munro J, Owen MJ, et al. Evidence for association between polymorphisms in the promoter and coding regions of the *5-HT2A* receptor gene and response to clozapine. *Mol Psychiatry.* 1998; 3:61–66.

Bumol TF, Watanabe AM. Genetic information, genomic technologies, and the future of drug discovery. *JAMA.* 2001; 285:551–555.

Cavazzana-Calvo M, Hacein-Bey S, de Saint Basile G, et al. Gene therapy of human severe combined immunodeficiency (SCID)-X1 disease. *Science.* 2000; 288:669–672.

Chan AWS, Chong KY, Martinovich C, Simerly C, Schatten G. Transgenic monkey produced by retroviral gene transfer into mature oocytes. *Science.* 2001; 291:309–312.

Collins FS, McKusick VA. Implications of the Human Genome Project for medical science. *JAMA.* 2001; 285:540–544.

Drysdale CM, McGraw DW, Stack CB, et al. Complex promoter and coding region beta 2-adrenergic receptor haplotypes alter receptor expression and predict in vivo responsiveness. *Proc Natl Acad Sci USA.* 2000; 97:10483–10488.

Evans WE, Relling MV. Pharmacogenomics: translating functional genomics into rational therapeutics. *Science.* 1999; 286:487–491.

Farlow MR, Lahiri DK, Poirier J, Davignon J, Hui S. Apolipoprotein E genotype and gender influence response to tacrine therapy. *Ann N Y Acad Sci.* 1996; 802:101–110.

Freed CR, Greene PE, Breeze RE, et al. Transplantation of embryonic dopamine neurons for severe Parkinson's disease. *N Engl J Med.* 2001; 344:710–719.

Gene therapy's trials. *Nature.* 2000; 405:599.

Grossman M, Raper SE, Kozarsky K, et al. Successful ex vivo gene therapy directed to liver in a patient with familial hypercholesterolaemia. *Nat Genet.* 1994; 6:335–341.

Higashi MK, Veenstra DL, Kondo LM, et al. Association between *CYP2C9* genetic variants and anticoagulation-related outcomes during warfarin therapy. *JAMA.* 2002; 287:1690–1698.

Human gene marker/therapy clinical protocols. *Hum Gene Ther.* 2000; 11:1745–1816.

Idle JR, Smith RL. Polymorphisms of oxidation at carbon centers of drugs and their clinical significance. *Drug Metab Rev.* 1979; 9:301–317.

Kaji EH, Leiden JM. Gene and stem cell therapies. *JAMA.* 2001; 285:545–550.

Kay MA, Manno CS, Ragni MV, et al. Evidence for gene transfer and expression of factor IX in haemophilia B patients treated with an AAV vector. *Nat Genet.* 2000; 24:257–261.

Kobinger GP, Weiner DJ, Yu Q-C, Wilson JM. Filovirus-pseudotyped lentiviral vector can efficiently and stably transduce airway epithelia in vivo. *Nat Biotechnol.* 2001; 19:225–230.

Lazarou J, Pomeranz BH, Corey PN. Incidence of adverse drug reactions in hospitalized patients: a meta-analysis of prospective studies. *JAMA.* 1998; 279:1200–1205.

May C, Rivella S, Callegari J, et al. Therapeutic haemoglobin synthesis in beta-thalassaemic mice expressing lentivirus-encoded human beta-globin. *Nature.* 2000; 406:82–86.

Meyer UA, Zanger UM. Molecular mechanisms of genetic polymorphisms of drug metabolism. *Annu Rev Pharmacol Toxicol.* 1997; 37:269–296.

Morgan JE. Cell and gene therapy in Duchenne muscular dystrophy. *Hum Gene Ther.* 1994; 5:165–173.

Nebert DW. Polymorphisms in drug-metabolizing enzymes: what is their clinical relevance and why do they exist? *Am J Hum Genet.* 1997; 60:265–271.

Poirier J, Delisle MC, Quirion R, et al. Apolipoprotein E4 allele as a predictor of cholinergic deficits and treatment outcome in Alzheimer's disease. *Proc Natl Acad Sci USA.* 1995; 92:12260–12264.

Pollard TD. The future of biomedical research: from the inventory of genes to understanding physiology and the molecular basis of disease. *JAMA.* 2002: 1725–1727.

Richard F, Helbecque N, Neuman E, Guez D, Levy R, Amouyel P. *APOE* genotyping and response to drug treatment in Alzheimer's disease. *Lancet.* 1997; 349(9051):539.

Seder RA, Gurunathan S. DNA vaccines—designer vaccines for the 21st century. *N Engl J Med.* 1999; 341:277–278.

Verlinsky Y, Rechitsky S, Verlinsky O, Masciangelo C, Lederer K, Kuliev A. Preimplantation diagnosis for early-onset Alzheimer's disease caused by *V717L* mutation. *JAMA.* 2002; 287:1018–1021.

Vile RG, Russell SJ, Lemoine NR. Cancer gene therapy: hard lessons and new courses. *Gene Ther.* 2000; 7:2–8.

Weiner DB, Kennedy RC. Genetic vaccines. *Sci Amer.* 1999; 281:50–57.

Useful Web Sites

Consensus statement overview: genetic testing for cystic fibrosis. Office of Disease Prevention/NIH Web site. Available at: http://odp.od.nih.gov/consensus/cons/106/106_intro.htm. Accessed August 6, 2002.

Editors' and Reporters' Guide to Biotechnology: Approved Biotechnology Drugs 1999. Biotechnology Industry Organization Web site. Available at: http://www.bio.org/aboutbio/drugs.html. Accessed August 6, 2002.

Frankel MS, Chapman AR for the American Association for the Advancement of Science. Human inheritable genetic modifications: assessing scientific, ethical, religious, and policy issues. 2000. Available at: http://www.aaas.org/spp/dspp/sfrl/germline/main.htm. Accessed August 6, 2002.

GeneTests Web site. Available at: http://www.genetests.org. Accessed August 6, 2002.

Genomics and Its Impact on Medicine and Society: A 2001 Primer. Department of Energy Web site. Available at: http://www.ornl.gov/hgmis/publicat/primer2001. Accessed August 6, 2002.

Human Genome Project information: DNA forensics. Department of Energy Web site. Available at: http://www.ornl.gov/hgmis/elsi/forensics.html. Accessed August 6, 2002.

Human Genome Project information: genetic disease information—*pronto!* Department of Energy Web site. Available at: http://www.ornl.gov/hgmis/medicine/assist.html. Accessed August 6, 2002.

Human Genome Project information: pharmacogenomics. Department of Energy Web site. Available at: http://www.ornl.gov/hgmis/medicine/pharma.html. Accessed August 6, 2002.

Medicines by design: the biological revolution in pharmacology. National Institutes of General Medicine Sciences/NIH Web site. Available at: http://www.nigms.nih.gov/news/science_ed/medbydes.html. Accessed August 6, 2002.

Medicines for you. National Institutes of General Medicine Sciences/NIH Web site. Available at: http://www.nigms.nih.gov/funding/medforyou.html. Accessed August 6, 2002.

National Coalition for Health Professional Education in Genetics (NCHPEG) Web site. Available at: http://www.nchpeg.org. Accessed August 6, 2002.

OMIM: Online Mendelian Inheritance in Man. National Center for Biotechnology Information/NIH Web site. Available at: http://www3.ncbi.nlm.nih.gov/Omim/. Accessed August 6, 2002.

Statement of the American Society of Clinical Oncology: genetic testing for cancer susceptibility. ASCO Web site. Available at: http://208.243.117.239/prof/pp/html/m_ppgenetc.htm. Accessed August 6, 2002.

U.S. Department of Health and Human Services. Understanding gene testing—a booklet from the National Institutes of Health. Access Excellence Web site. Available at: http://www.accessexcellence.org/AE/AEPC/NIH/index.html. Accessed August 6, 2002.

Weiner DB, Kennedy RC. Genetic vaccines. *Sci Amer.* 1999; 281:50–57. Available at: http://www.sciam.com. Accessed December 26, 2001.

6

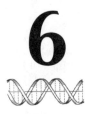

Genetics and Nutrition Therapy

As we saw in Chapter 5, significant progress is being made in applying genetic research to medical therapy. Nutrition professionals will soon be expected to have a working knowledge of these medical applications as they become commonplace, from DNA-based diagnostic testing to gene therapy. We will continue to play a valuable support role through our ability to extend the services of the health care team, from being able to take and analyze extensive family histories to being able to help patients as they explore the complex genetic options available to them.

ON THE HORIZON: GENE-BASED NUTRITION THERAPY

As the direct linkages among genes, proteins, disease, and nutritional modifiers become known, nutrition professionals will be expected to help clients make sense of the often bewildering information available to them and to help them sort through the options. We will also need to be able to use this information to develop disease management and disease prevention strategies for clients.

Where Are We Headed?

The genetics-savvy nutrition professional will play an increasingly pivotal role on the health care team. Ultimately, clients will come to us with their genotypes in hand. The medical therapies they are undergoing will be gene-based. Nutrition professionals of the future will have a deeper understanding of what is wrong with the client and what the physician's treatment goals are specifically targeting. We will also be able to convert genotypes into effective outcomes through gene-based nutrition therapy and will be the primary sources of information for how food and dietary supplements interact with particular genotypes. Gene-based nutrition therapy will be the key to preventive health. Our challenge will be to understand what the genotype is telling us in terms of which diseases the client is susceptible to and their projected severity based on the particular genetic variant the client has. We will need to know which nutrition and other lifestyle choices will best prevent, or at least minimize the impact of, the diseases to which the client is susceptible.

Additionally, the genetics-savvy nutrition professional will be able to fill a growing gap in the need for health care professionals with genetics knowledge who also have counseling skills. Being alert to the diseases that are expressed in the client's extended family will become an increasingly important tool in preventing disease development. Knowing how those diseases are inherited, how they present early on, and which family members are likely to be susceptible will be a valuable skill that the nutrition professional brings to the health care team and a valuable contribution to the overall health management of clients and their families.

Why go to all the trouble to customize nutrition therapy to one's genes? "Everyone knows" that a high-complex-carbohydrate, low-fat, low-sodium diet with lots of fruits and vegetables will take care of most chronic disease risk. Some people won't need all that precaution, but it won't hurt them to live that way, will it? Why not just give everyone at risk for, say, type 2 diabetes, the same weight management/blood glucose management/blood pressure management/antiatherogenesis diet? For one thing, we know there are at least 150 different genotypes that all give rise to type 2 diabetes of varying severity, that people respond differently to low-fat diets depending on their genotype (for some, such diets are actually atherogenic), and that not everyone has salt-responsive hypertension. Second, it's a quality of life issue. Life is too short to spend it counting calories, carbohydrates, saturated fat, and sodium grams if your genotype doesn't require this approach. Your type 2 diabetes may be due to a genotype that responds to a high-carbohydrate diet with weight gain, which triggers the metabolic syndrome that ultimately leads to type 2 diabetes. For you, the appropriate therapy is simply to adjust the macronutrient content of the diet to support normal weight maintenance. When this adjustment is made, the impaired glucose tolerance, hypertension, and risk of atherosclerosis may no longer be an issue.

Where Are We Now?

Genes underlie all metabolic and physiologic function. Nutrition, as we'll see, is a primary influencer of these outcomes. The promise for gene-based nutrition therapy is, therefore, enormous. However, practical applications of genetic research to nutrition therapy lag behind those of medical therapy. Why is this?

There are several reasons. The direct connection between nutrition and health is not yet fully appreciated, which has limited our thinking as well as the push for clinical studies. Genetics is just now being recognized as central to medicine. Not surprisingly, recognition of its connections to nutrition lags even further behind. There needs to be a major shift in thinking concerning the role of diet and dietary supplements to the functioning of the body. Second, nutrition's primary challenges today concern the chronic diseases. There are enormous gaps in our understanding of these diseases, including the gene/function association for each. Considerably more basic science research is needed before the full impact of genetic applications to nutrition therapy will be evident.

These major limitations aside, there is still much that we can be doing to launch gene-based nutrition therapy. First, we can recognize the primary role that genetics plays in the extensive variation in client response to nutrition therapy. This realization alone will change our approach to nutrition therapy and counseling. Second, we can develop the mindset that underneath even the most complex condition is an orderly gene/protein/function relationship that can be sorted out and that almost always can be influenced in some way by nutrition, either directly or indirectly. We just don't know what these relationships are as yet. Third, we can begin now to formulate a framework for how nutrition influences genetic outcomes and use this framework to guide us in converting basic science into practical applications as this field develops.

RETHINKING NUTRITION THERAPY FROM A GENETIC PERSPECTIVE

Every practicing nutrition professional knows the frustration of encountering a wide spectrum of therapeutic responses to nutritional therapies, even in the most motivated clients. What we're encountering here is the impact of genetic variation on therapeutic response. This heterogeneity has long been seen with cardiovascular disease, obesity, type 2 diabetes, and cancer, but we've looked for answers in many places before realizing that the unique genetic makeup of each individual is undercutting our therapeutic approaches. Just as pharmacologists are beginning to use genetic profiling to target drugs to drug responders/nonresponders to maximize the therapeutic benefits and minimize the adverse effects, so nutrition professionals will need to target food and dietary supplements to genetic profiles. The next era in nutrition therapy will be the era of nutritional genomics, using gene-directed dietary choices to prevent and ameliorate disease.

Nutrition and Genetic Outcomes

That we can influence the outcome of our genes is a revolutionary idea and an exciting one! What's even more exciting for nutrition professionals is the emerging realization that nutrition is going to be a major player in the new approach to keeping people healthy. The old idea that genetics is deterministic and that humans are simply the product of their genes has given way to the realization that genes establish our upper and lower functional potentials. It's environmental factors that determine where within that potential we actually function. Environmental factors include infectious, chemical, physical, nutritional, and behavioral factors, of which nutritional factors are possibly the most powerful in terms of altering the impact that the message in our genes actually has on our lives. For example, we'll never be able to run any faster nor jump any higher than our body mechanics permit, but, given these genetically determined physiological limits, where on the continuum will we actually fall? Here's where lifestyle choices come in. With top-quality training and nutrition we can function at the upper limits of our potential, or we can choose to eat poorly, not train, and likely fall far short of our maximum potential as a result.

For most health care professionals, genetics has been thought of as being responsible for severe, usually incurable, diseases such as cystic fibrosis, Huntington's disease, Tay-Sachs, and sickle cell disease. These disorders are caused by mutations in single genes, which lead to dysfunction in the proteins produced by those genes, which in turn leads to health problems. With these disorders there's a clear correlation between the mutation and the development of the disease. The occurrence of any one disease may be rare, but, collectively, single-gene disorders are not rare and have contributed substantially to our understanding of the direct connection between genetics and disease.

What we're now realizing is that change in the DNA base composition of the genetic material is the normal consequence of ongoing evolution within a species and that genetic variation between individuals not only is common—it's what makes us uniquely ourselves. We see the bigger picture; we just don't yet have the details as to which variations confer susceptibility to which diseases.

Even less well understood is which environmental factors influence each of these susceptibility genes and exactly how that interaction occurs. Complicating the situation still further is the likelihood that many chronic diseases may well turn out to be multigenic (influenced by more than one gene) and multifactorial (with environmental as well as genetic factors having an influence). These diseases will be more difficult to sort out mechanistically than the single-gene disorders, but it's just a matter of time given the speed at which our understanding of the genetic basis of disease is progressing.

Disease as a Genetic-Based Condition

The important concept for health care professionals to realize is that "genetic disease" is not a separate category of disease. Virtually all disease is genetic in origin, even infectious disease. The infectious agent is not a genetic factor per se, but its ability to penetrate the human body and reproduce to a high enough titer to have a pathological effect is directly related to the genetic makeup of the human being it is invading. Rather than genetic disease being a distinct entity, we must acknowledge the genetic underpinning of all human functioning, whether it results in good health or ill health, and begin thinking of disease in terms of a spectrum of causes that range from totally genetic on one end to totally environmental on the other. We need to begin thinking about the interaction of genetic susceptibility and environmental factors, particularly nutrition.

In some cases, as with gluten-sensitive enteropathy (GSE), nutrition can completely change the health outcome of someone who is genetically susceptible. If individuals with GSE avoid gluten-containing foods, they will be functionally normal and phenotypically indistinguishable from someone who does not carry this mutation. They will develop this syndrome only if they do not match their food to their genes. Their genes have not changed, but their health outcomes have dramatically changed as a result of their nutrition choices.

Thus, health is a dynamic balance between normal and pathological processes—between function and dysfunction—and there are various points at which conscious choice can skew this balance in one direction or the other. Where we function on our personal health continuum is directly related to the interaction between the susceptibilities encoded in our genes and our lifestyle choices, which include the foods we eat, the air we breathe, where we live, the thoughts we think, whether or not we're physically active, and so on. As nutrition professionals we can have enormous influence on people as to whether their choices support the wellness or the illness end of their personal health continuum. As we learn more about which nutrients influence which genes, we can translate that information into personal health strategies that will maximize each person's unique genetic potential. No doubt, nutritional genomics is uncharted territory, but it's an uncharted territory through which nutrition professionals are well suited to serve as guides.

THE GENETICS-NUTRITION CONNECTION

Nutrition therapy is changing from an emphasis on food per se to a focus on what molecules foods contain and how those molecules are used by the cells in the body. From a cell's perspective, a meal of roast chicken, rice pilaf, green beans, milk, and fresh strawberries represents a supply of amino acids, fatty acids, starch, fiber, and a variety of vitamins, minerals, and phytonutrients, essentially all the end products of digestion. These foods ultimately serve as sources of the components used in the body's many reactions and as therapeutic agents that can fill biochemical gaps caused by faulty genes, influence cellular activities such as membrane function and enzyme action, or affect the cell more fundamentally by turning genes on or off or fine-tuning the magnitude of their expression.

The Role of Genes

Genes underlie each of the life-sustaining activities of cells, and the products of the genes–proteins–are what carry out the actual work. Genes must be expressed in order to make proteins. If there's an error in a gene, it may affect the function of the protein coded for by that gene. The environment in which an organism lives determines the proteins needed for that organism to survive and function optimally. Environmental factors, such as nutrients, send signals to the genetic information communicating the need to turn on or off certain genetic segments and the proteins they encode. To the cell, nutrients serve as information about the surrounding environment, and the cell responds accordingly. The key to using nutrition to influence genetic outcomes lies in what the various proteins in the cell do, how nutrition is involved in these activities, how a change in a gene affects the production or function of a protein, and how nutrition can influence these potentially negative outcomes.

The Role of Proteins

Proteins are fundamental to cells. They serve as enzymes, receptors, carriers and transporters, blood-clotting proteins, structural and contractile proteins, and as hormones and other messenger molecules. A key goal of preventive health care is to keep all these gene-derived proteins functioning optimally and to provide solutions when dysfunction occurs. Nutrition is an essential tool because it provides the raw materials for the synthesis and function of these proteins, but nutrition can also compensate for limitations in the genetic information. We're familiar with the concept of essential nutrients: amino acids, fatty acids, vitamins, and minerals that human beings are unable to synthesize and that must, therefore, be provided by the diet. What we may not be familiar with is the fact that many of these commonplace requirements are examples of nutrition compensating for limitations in our genes. Evolution has left the human species with mutations that make us unable to produce critical enzymes needed for synthesizing vitamins such as vitamin C and several essential amino acids and fatty acids. In earlier times humankind may not have understood which genes were mutated and which enzymes were thereby absent or dysfunctional, but people rapidly learned that failure to eat certain foods that supplied these nutrients (which they identified through trial and error) resulted in disease and, often, death. Those foods came from species that did not have the same mutations as human beings and therefore could supply the missing components, so disease was prevented. Now we understand that mutations are responsible for our inability to make these essential nutrients. By supplying these substances through nutrition, we circumvent the disease susceptibility encoded in our genes.

The Role of Nutrition

By compensating for the effects of faulty proteins, nutrition is a powerful tool for managing, correcting, and preventing genetic susceptibility to health impairment. In addition to circumventing lethal events, nutrition can compensate for a condition that has a less dramatic impact on health.

For example, a mutation in the genetic information coding for a particular enzyme in a metabolic pathway can cause the activity of a protein to be too low to supply the level of a needed metabolite. Judicious supplementation with either the end product metabolite itself or an intermediary metabolite further downstream in the metabolic pathway essentially "wires around" the defective enzyme's inability to produce the intermediate, as in the case of the essential nutrients discussed in the previous paragraph. For proteins that are membrane receptors, mutations in the genetic material can affect the structure of that protein so that its ability to recognize its ligand or fit properly into the cell membrane is decreased. Enriching the diet with omega-3 fatty acids, for example, can improve the fluidity of the lipid bilayer membrane and improve receptor function.

Alternatively, nutrition may act directly at the level of gene expression by decreasing or increasing the transcription of a particular gene into messenger RNA or the translation of a particular messenger RNA into protein. For example, when the liver has a greater than normal level of toxic molecules to detoxify, as can occur when an individual is taking several medications at once, undergoing chemotherapy, or exposed to everyday toxic chemicals, increased activity of the liver detoxification enzymes is needed. The glucosinolates in broccoli, cauliflower, brussels sprouts, and other cruciferous vegetables can increase gene expression of a key detoxification enzyme, which in turn helps reduce the toxic load by converting the toxin into a product that can be excreted. In this case phytonutrients from the cruciferous vegetables are critical for preventing the health damage that these toxic agents can cause, and they achieve their effect by increasing gene expression.

Nutrition, then, is arguably *the* most powerful tool for influencing genetic susceptibility. It has the ability to fill biochemical gaps created by mistakes in the genetic information that, left unfilled, lead to disease and death. It also has the ability to influence gene expression. Various examples, likely to be encountered in practice, of how nutrition plays this important role are discussed subsequently in this chapter. However, the interaction between genes and environmental factors such as nutrition is complex and, presently, we understand few of the details of how environmental factors influence genetic susceptibility. It's important, therefore, to develop a conceptual framework that can be filled in over time as the details become known. One logical framework is offered here. What you'll rapidly realize is that, for conditions where considerable knowledge is available about the disease process and the genes and proteins involved, these conditions fit neatly into the framework. Our understanding of the chronic diseases, however, is still a muddle, and it's far more difficult to find a place for them within any framework. Be patient. With the increasing sophistication of thinking and technology directed at the gene-protein-environment-health puzzle, the fundamentals underlying chronic diseases will ultimately surface.

COMPENSATING FOR GENETIC LIMITATIONS

A helpful framework for thinking about how nutrition will be used to compensate for genetic limitations is to think in terms of nutrition doing the following:

- Compensating for a faulty protein
- Influencing gene expression to compensate for the environment in which the organism finds itself

There may be other gene-nutrient interactions that will surface in time, but this framework provides a solid foundation for beginning to think about nutrition from a new perspective.

Compensating for a Faulty Protein

For mutations that lead to defective proteins, the primary anticipated applications of nutrition therapy include providing needed metabolites and preventing potentially harmful events. Nutrition can supplement the low levels of metabolites produced by faulty enzymes or, in the case of totally dysfunctional enzymes, potentially serve as the sole source of the needed metabolites. Nutrition can also supply cofactors for which the mutant protein has a reduced affinity, requiring much higher levels of cofactors to support the function of that protein. Where the mutation results in an accumulation of a potentially toxic intermediate, the goal of nutrition therapy is to reduce the concentration of the toxin. For proteins other than metabolic enzymes, the aim of nutrition therapy may be to prevent a harmful reaction or compensate for a faulty receptor or hormone.

Preventing a deficiency of a necessary metabolite   A common situation in which a metabolite is supplied in too low a concentration to fill the needs of the cells results from the action of a defective cellular component such as a metabolic enzyme, a transporter or carrier, or a receptor. The protein is defective and unable to bind to its ligand (its substrate or a required coenzyme factor) and carry out its normal activity. Metabolic enzymes fail to convert enough of one metabolite into another, transporters fail to move sufficient amounts of nutrients from one compartment to another, or hormones fail to convey the signal needed for downstream events to take place. The end result is a cellular handicap that can range from mild to severe and even lethal.

Two strategic approaches that can be taken involve

1. Supplying the needed metabolite
2. Increasing the effectiveness of the defective protein

The first approach is straightforward. There are numerous examples in which loss of function of an enzyme results in a requirement for a metabolic end product that, if left unsupplied, leads to negative health consequences. Examples familiar to nutrition professionals include the mutations in the human genome that make us unable to produce the essential nutrients, as previously discussed, which we supply in the diet to compensate for these biochemical gaps. Beyond these genetic limitations that all of us share, individuals have specific mutations that can lead to disease. An error in any gene coding for any of the thousands of enzymes involved in the systematic conversion of one metabolite into another provides an instance of this type of compensation. Once the metabolic pathway is known and the metabolites available, it becomes possible to supply the missing metabolite through food or targeted supplementation and alleviate the biochemical problem caused by the faulty gene. This approach is straightforward and can be applied to virtually any metabolic enzyme deficiency that results from a genetic defect.

The second approach of using nutrition to improve the activity of a protein is also straightforward in theory but not yet commonly used. Typically in biochemistry, the affinity of an enzyme for its substrate is measured in terms of its Michaelis-Menten constant (K_m). The lower the affinity, the higher the K_m, and the higher the concentration of substrate that's needed for the reaction to proceed at a normal rate. Because of genetic mutations and resulting polymorphism, the same enzyme isolated from different people can vary considerably in its affinity for its substrate. Similarly, for those enzymes that have coenzyme factors, such as one of the vitamins, genetic changes can result in altered affinities of the enzyme protein for its cofactor. For these defective proteins to work, higher than normal concentrations of substrate or cofactor must be provided. In many cases these required concentrations well exceed the recommended intake levels. Ames and colleagues published a well considered review of this concept in the *American Journal of Clinical Nutrition,* providing numerous examples of gene-based nutrition considerations that lead to the need for high-dose vitamin therapy.

Similarly, proteins serve as receptors and transporters embedded within the membranes that surround cells and subcellular organelles, such as the nucleus and mitochondrion. As an example, a mutation in the insulin receptor can lead to glucose intolerance and its accompanying sequelae. Although studies here are not definitive, various nutritional interventions are being used to try to compensate for the receptor's impaired function. Among the approaches are the use of chromium dietary supplements to improve binding at the insulin receptor and omega-3 fatty acids to help indirectly by increasing cells' membrane fluidity and improving receptor-ligand interactions. Another approach is to try to mimic the insulin receptor action with the use of dietary supplements, such as vanadyl sulfate, thereby circumventing the limitations of the dysfunctional receptor. Additionally, exercise appears to increase availability of the glucose translocator proteins, which may circumvent the problem as well. The genetic defect remains, but nutrition and other lifestyle approaches offer options for working around the limitations. It's this type of thinking that's going on in laboratories around the world to develop nutrition as a useful tool for modifying genetic outcomes.

Preventing an excess of a toxic metabolite   Commonly the loss of an enzyme in a metabolic pathway results not only in a missing end product but also in an accumulation of another metabolite that can be toxic. Such is the case with phenylketonuria (PKU), which results from a mutation in the enzyme phenylalanine hydroxylase, which is needed to convert phenylalanine to the amino acid tyrosine. People with this disorder must obtain tyrosine from their diet, but they also need to reduce the phenylalanine content of the diet to prevent it from building up and being metabolized to another intermediate, phenylpyruvate. Excess phenylpyruvate is toxic to developing neural tissue and leads to mental retardation if left unchecked. This disorder is readily amenable to nutritional therapy, but it must be detected early and a low-phenylalanine diet begun soon after birth to prevent the neurological damage.

Other examples of disorders of amino acid metabolism that result in toxic accumulation include homocystinuria and maple syrup urine disease (MSUD). In the latter, individuals cannot decarboxylate the alpha-ketoacids formed from the branched-chain amino acids leucine, valine, and isoleucine. The alpha-ketoacids accumulate and cause neurodegeneration and death in the first few months of life. The disease is so named because the urine of affected people smells like maple syrup. Dietary intervention at this time involves a delicate balance of keeping the branched-chain amino acid content of the diet low and still keeping protein levels high enough to support growth and development. The defective enzyme is branched-chain alpha-ketoacid decarboxylase, a multimeric enzyme encoded by six genes. A defect in any of these genes can result in MSUD. As our knowledge increases, it will likely turn out that mutations in the various genes are associated with different severities of MSUD. Perhaps some mutations will respond to particular nutritional interventions, such as the ability of a nutrient to improve the conformation or assembly of the enzyme complex and, thereby, the function of the enzyme.

Homocystinuria has gained prominence in recent years because it pointed to elevated blood homocysteine levels as an independent risk factor in heart disease. Homocystinuria is the result of a mutation in the gene that codes for cystathionine beta synthase, with the result that homocysteine cannot be converted to the amino acid cysteine. Homocysteine accumulates and is thought to irritate the endothelial lining of the blood vessels and set the stage for atherosclerosis, which in turn leads to cardiovascular disease and its complications. Once again, dietary therapy can compensate for the genetic limitation. In the presence of adequate levels of folate and B_{12} and the dietary supplement betaine (trimethylglycine), homocysteine can be converted to methionine and other nontoxic metabolites, which decreases homocysteine levels and the attendant cardiovascular risk.

Homocystinuria is a rare disorder. Far more common are two polymorphisms for the enzyme 5-methyltetrahydrofolate reductase (MTHFR). This enzyme catalyzes the conversion of 5,10-methylenetetrahydrofolate to 5-methyltetrahydrofolate, the predominant form of folate in plasma and the methyl donor for the methylation of homocysteine to form methionine. One polymorphism involves the mutation C677T (replacement of the DNA base cytosine, C, by thymine, T, at base pair number 677). The genetic change results in an amino acid change in the MTHFR protein, with valine replacing alanine. The enzyme is thermolabile and has reduced activity. The second polymorphism involves the A1298C mutation, in which cytosine has replaced adenine, A, at base pair 1298, which results in a substitution of the amino acid alanine for glutamate in the MTHFR enzyme. When individuals who have two copies of the defective C677T mutation (designated T/T) also have impaired folate status, mild hyperhomocysteinemia results. Typically, increasing the folate concentration decreases homocysteine levels. An interesting question that has not been resolved is whether such individuals require greater than the standard recommendation of 400 micrograms of folate per day. The A1298C mutation, even in the homozygous C/C state, is not associated with elevated plasma homocysteine. Clearly the nutritional therapy would differ for individuals depending on which mutation in the MTHFR gene they had and, if they were homozygous for the C677T mutation, whether they were sufficient for folate nutriture.

Galactosemia is a disorder of carbohydrate metabolism and another example of a metabolic enzyme defect that results in toxic metabolite accumulation. In the case of galactosemia, the enzyme galactose-1-phosphate uridyl transferase is defective, and galactose cannot be converted to glucose. Galactose accumulates in the blood and is either reduced to galactitol or oxidized to galactonate. By mechanisms not fully understood, one or both of these metabolites is harmful. Restricting the diet in galactose reduces the morbidity associated with this disease. A future nutritional approach might be to determine whether nutrients could increase gene expression of enzymes that could convert galactitol and galactonate into harmless intermediates, thereby circumventing the negative outcomes of this genetic defect.

Lactose intolerance, an inability to metabolize the milk sugar lactose, results from insufficient lactase enzyme being produced in the small intestine. The sugar is not cleaved into its glucose and galactose components, which would normally be absorbed in the small intestine, but instead is metabolized by the bacteria that live in the intestines. Individuals typically experience considerable gas, bloating, and generalized discomfort when they eat foods containing lactose. This condition may result from a genetic defect in lactase production or in the lactase gene, or it may be secondary to conditions that disrupt the function of the small intestine where lactase is produced. One solution is to avoid lactose-containing foods and medications. Another is to use specially treated, lactose-free foods to reduce the concentration of lactose ingested. Alternatively, replacement lactase can be provided as a dietary supplement so that lactose can be metabolized and the symptoms avoided. A novel approach is to genetically engineer one of the strains of "friendly" bacteria (probiotics) that reside in the small intestine so that the bacteria can cleave lactose into glucose and galactose, which can then be absorbed. Individuals with lactase limitations could enjoy dairy products without the complications of digestive upset or needing to resort to special foods or supplements.

Preventing a toxic event As discussed briefly earlier in this chapter, gluten-sensitive enteropathy (GSE) is an excellent example of how nutrition can alter genetic outcomes. Foods containing gluten, such as wheat, barley, rye, and certain components derived from them, cause an inflammatory response in the small intestinal mucosa, which can lead to a major disruption of nutrient absorption and increased intestinal permeability. Nutrition therapy, in the form of elimination of gluten from the diet, prevents the toxic reaction and allows such individuals to appear phenotypically normal even though their genes carry the susceptibility for disease.

Hemochromatosis, also called iron overload disease, is another example of a toxic event that can be circumvented with early intervention. Alterations in at least one gene and possibly others lead to increased absorption of iron from the intestinal tract. The excess iron can result in hepatic fibrosis, diabetes mellitus, and cardiac failure. Although medical therapy is the primary therapy, limiting iron intake from the diet and dietary supplements should be considered. Including high levels of antioxidants from food and dietary supplements may be another important aspect of nutrition therapy, because iron is a pro-oxidant and free-radical-mediated damage is a major concern with excess iron.

Like gluten-sensitive enteropathy, hemochromatosis is quite common (approximately one individual in 250 to 400 is homozygous; one in eight to ten is heterozygous) but often goes undiagnosed for years. A genetics-savvy nutrition professional can be valuable here. Knowing that these disorders are common, the nutrition professional will be alert to their early signs and, understanding their genetic transmission, will be able to identify those family members at highest risk and assist in obtaining early intervention for these individuals.

Hereditary fructose intolerance is another example of preventing phenotypic expression of a genotype that can cause a toxic situation. A deficiency of fructose-1,6-biphosphate aldolase leads to inability to metabolize fructose. Symptoms are typically seen in infants after weaning and include poor feeding, failure to thrive, and ultimately liver and kidney damage and death. Individuals are asymptomatic, however, unless they eat fructose or sucrose, a compound of glucose and fructose.

Influencing Gene Expression

Nutrients can increase or decrease gene expression directly through their effects on DNA-binding proteins that control transcription or indirectly through effects on translation initiation or post-translational processing. In transcriptional control, regulation is at the level of DNA's conversion into messenger RNA and involves nutrients interacting with transcriptional factors that in turn interact with the DNA and promote or inhibit RNA polymerase enzymes from transcribing the DNA into messenger RNA.

With translation initiation or post-translational processing, control is at the level of translating the message into protein. Regulation of gene expression by controlling translation initiation involves increasing or decreasing the assembly of an intact ribosome on which the message is translated into a protein. Control at the level of post-translational processing involves preventing the modifications that occur to a protein following its synthesis, such as cleavage of the pro-form into the active form or adding sugar residues to form glycoproteins.

Direct influence on gene expression   The most common known interaction of nutrients with the genetic material occurs through their ability to bind to DNA-binding proteins known as transcription factors. A variety of transcription factors exist and are known to interact with the regulatory regions of a gene and promote or inhibit gene expression. Virtually all of the work to date has been done with cultured cells or other in vitro systems.

It is speculated that, early in evolution, organisms had a need to sense changes in the nutrient environment and so developed nutrient-regulated switches for gene expression, much like a primitive hormonal signaling system. As organisms evolved into more complex beings, nutrients continued to be an effective signaling mechanism for turning gene expression on and off in response to the environment. The nutrients themselves do not bind directly to DNA but instead bind to a transcription element, such as PPARs, HNF4 alpha, NF kappa B, or SREBP1c.

One fairly well-characterized example of the interaction among transcription factors and nutrients is the PPAR (peroxisome proliferator-activated receptor) family, which is a set of lipid-activated transcription factors, proteins that are influenced by essential fatty acids in the diet. Much of this work has been reported by Steven Clarke and associates at the University of Texas at Austin (Clarke, 1999; Clarke et al., 1999; Jump and Clarke, 1999; Price et al., 2000; Clarke, 2001; Teran-Garcia et al., 2002). The PPAR protein has two binding sites: one for the ligand that will activate it (fatty acids) and another for binding to a second transcription factor, the retinoid receptor Xalpha (Xα, also called RXRα). Together the PPAR and Xalpha transcription factors form a dimer, which then binds to the DNA in the regulatory region upstream from the start signal of the genes whose expression is regulated by these transcription factors. Among the genes known to be regulated by PPAR are several that are involved in the oxidation and synthesis of lipids, cellular differentiation, and membrane receptor expression. Polyunsaturated fatty acids, particularly the omega-3 and omega-6 series, bind to the various PPAR transcription factors and activate them. The expression of the various genes that are under the regulation of the PPAR transcription factors is strongly influenced by the fatty acid composition of the diet. Defining the specifics of PPARs, fatty acids, and gene expression will result in new approaches by which the foods and dietary supplements we take in can be used to effect a desired genetic response.

Other examples of nutrients interacting with transcription factors to promote gene expression include the following:

- Omega-3 fatty acids and genes that control lipid oxidation in liver and skeletal muscle (carnitine palmitoyltransferase-1 and acyl CoA oxidase, for example)
- Zinc and the metallothionein 1, zinc transporter 2, cholecystokinin, and uroguanylin genes
- Conjugated linoleic acid and increased expression of genes controlled by the transcription factor peroxisome proliferator-activated receptor alpha (PPARα)
- Glucosinolates and increased gene expression of the glutathione enzymes involved in phase II detoxification
- Carotenoids and increased expression of the connexin 43 gene in chemoprevention
- Increased expression of the CD36 receptor protein on the surface of macrophages (scavenger pathway for modified LDL-C) through the interaction of oxidized LDL-C and the transcription factor peroxisome proliferator-activated receptor gamma (PPARγ).

Nutrients can also interact with transcription factors to turn off gene expression. Examples of the negative influence of nutrients on gene expression include the following:

- Omega-3 fatty acids and sterol regulatory element binding protein-1 (SREBP-1)
- The flavonoid quercetin and the expression of androgen-responsive genes implicated in the development and progression of prostate cancer

- Genistein (soy isoflavone) and its interference with nuclear factor-kappa B transcription factor induction of androgen-sensitive gene expression in prostate cancer cells
- Antioxidant nutrients, ranging from N-acetyl L-cysteine to various flavonoids, have been shown to suppress gene expression induced by inflammatory responses
- Conjugated linoleic acid and stearoyl-CoA desaturase 1 gene in adipocytes
- Indole-3-carbinol and CYPB1B, which metabolizes the estrogen metabolite estrone to the carcinogen 4-hydroxyestrone.

Indirect influence on gene expression through translation initiation
Nutrients that appear to decrease translation initiation include the following:

- Amino acids that, when insufficient, decrease translation initiation so that messenger RNA translation decreases
- The furanocoumarins in grapefruit and the decreased translation of intestinal CYP450 3A4 mRNA.

THE CHALLENGE OF THE CHRONIC DISEASES

The prevalent chronic diseases, such as cancer, cardiovascular disease, type 2 diabetes, hypertension, inflammatory bowel disorders, neurological disorders, obesity, and osteoporosis, are complex conditions. They are thought to result from multiple genes (multigenic), multiple environmental factors (multifactorial), or a combination of the two. In no case have the genes or the environmental factors been fully identified, but the types of questions that are being asked have an impact on how these diseases will ultimately be approached nutritionally:

- Which genes are associated with which diseases and, within these genes, which DNA sequence variations influence disease susceptibility? (There is likely to be a continuum, a gradient of effects of genetic variation on function, that correlates with the specific region of DNA that is altered.)
- More specifically, how do these variations influence the sensitivity of an individual to environmental influences?
- How does diet affect each of these genes and their variants? Can diet increase or decrease susceptibility to disease? Which nutrients can do so, and how?

Progress in sorting through the many genes and environmental factors involved is likely to be slow. It may be that some or all of these disorders are phenotypically similar but genotypically distinct, in much the same way that cancer is a heterogeneous collection of disorders. It's not possible to review here the details of each chronic disease, but it is helpful from a framework standpoint to be aware of some of the questions that have already surfaced about these diseases, and the types of answers that are likely to be sought over the next five to ten years. The major focus will be to identify associations of genes with medical conditions, to clarify the effects of the various alleles (variants) on the severity of the condition, to identify the proteins coded for by the normal and mutant variants and associate them with the different phenotypes, and to customize medical and nutritional therapies based on this information.

Cardiovascular Disease

As the number-one killer in the United States, cardiovascular disease is a fitting example of how genetic information can be used to tailor therapeutic approaches. This chronic disorder is multigenic and multifactorial. The key point with cardiovascular disease is that we know there is wide variability in individual levels of LDL-cholesterol and HDL-cholesterol, extent of dietary cholesterol absorption in response to dietary fat, and serum cholesterol response to lowering the fat in the diet. Genetic variation is almost certainly the underlying cause, but we don't yet know which genetic variations correspond to which responses. This information will form the basis for developing therapeutic approaches, both medical/pharmacological and nutritional.

Among the more promising gene-diet interactions that are known are the dietary responses of individuals with variants in the genes that code for the plasma apolipoproteins, which are a family of lipid-binding proteins that regulate lipoprotein metabolism within the vascular system. Many of these genes are polymorphic, and considerable data have been generated for the apo A-I, apo A-IV, apo B-100, and apo E lipoproteins with respect to their involvement in the physiological response to diet.

Apo A-I is the primary lipoprotein of HDL. Genetic variants (differing alleles) have been described in which individuals with these alleles remove cholesterol from cells more effectively than people with the normal variant do and are resistant to heart disease despite the presence of other risk factors. Diet and lifestyle counseling for individuals with one of these genetic variants would focus more on minimizing the other risk factors rather than on lowering saturated fat and increasing HDL levels. Conversely, those with apo A-I alleles that lead to decreased function of HDL-cholesterol are at increased risk of heart disease and need to watch their dietary fat intake closely (Schaefer et al., 1982). As an aside, promising studies with transgenic mice that overexpress the human *APOA-I* gene (normal variant) have shown an increase in HDL and a decrease in atherosclerotic lesions, which suggests that gene therapy may eventually be an option for apo A-I defects (Benoit et al., 1999).

Apolipoprotein A-IV is synthesized by the small intestine during fat absorption and binds dietary fat. The *APOA-IV* gene has two known alleles, *IV-1* and *IV-2*, with the *IV-1* allele being the normal variant. In studies that examined the impact of these two alleles on the individual's ability to control blood lipid levels in response to dietary cholesterol intake, it has been observed that the *IV-2* allele positively affects the response of plasma cholesterol concentration, both total cholesterol and LDL-cholesterol (McCombs et al., 1994). Eggs were chosen as the source of dietary cholesterol, and the experimental group consumed four egg yolks per day. Those homozygous for the *IV-1* allele (*A-IV-1/1*) had significantly elevated plasma total cholesterol and LDL-cholesterol levels, whereas heterozygotes (those with the one copy of the *IV-1* allele and one copy of the *IV-2* allele) had minimally elevated plasma cholesterol, which suggests that the *IV-2* allele blunts the hypercholesterolemic response. No changes were observed with either genotype with respect to triglycerides or HDL-C. Because the carrier rate in the United States for the *IV-2* allele is estimated to be one in seven, knowing the *A-IV* allele status of an individual would be helpful in tailoring advice concerning dietary fat intake.

Apolipoprotein B-100 is the chief protein component of LDL. Functioning as the ligand between the LDL-cholesterol molecule and the LDL receptor, it facilitates removal of LDL-cholesterol from circulation. Mutations in the apolipoprotein B gene or the LDL receptor affect the binding of LDL-cholesterol to the receptor and lead to elevated plasma LDL-cholesterol levels. Typically the cholesterol level is quite high and necessitates pharmacological management as the primary strategy, but it's likely that alleles exist that have less extreme effects, which might be managed with diet.

The density of the LDL particle and its relationship to atherogenesis is leading to biochemical and genetic laboratory analyses that predict susceptibility to cardiovascular disease. The relationship between LDL density and atherogenesis has been studied for many years by Krauss and colleagues at

Lawrence Berkeley National Laboratory and by Superko and coworkers, now at Berkeley HeartLab (Austin et al., 1990; Nishini, 1992; Krauss, 1994, Dreon et al., 1994; Superko et al., 1997; Dreon et al., 2000). These workers have characterized the LDL particle in reference to its use as a predictor of cardiovascular disease susceptibility, its prevalence, and its response to diet and drugs.

Density of the LDL particle is a heritable trait, sometimes called "small LDL trait." As measured in an analytical ultracentrifuge, LDL occurs in one of two density patterns: large and buoyant, called subclass pattern A, or small and dense, called subclass pattern B. Small, dense LDL particles are associated with atherogenesis. Large, buoyant LDL particles, pattern A, are not. Pattern B is accompanied by elevated triglycerides, reduced HDL and apo A-1, and insulin resistance. By fractionating the LDL into multiple subclasses, it appears possible to detect who is susceptible to developing heart disease.

The smaller the peak LDL particle diameter, the greater the risk. When other risk factors are present, such as elevated apo B-100 or fasting insulin or a combination of risk factors, cardiovascular disease susceptibility increases significantly (Lamarche et al., 1997; Lamarche et al., 1998).

Dreon and coworkers have investigated the effect of a low-fat diet on LDL particle size (Dreon et al., 1994; Dreon et al., 1995; Dreon et al., 2000). Although atherogenic pattern B individuals respond with lowered LDL-cholesterol and a reduction in apo B, pattern A individuals convert from the nonatherogenic large, buoyant LDL particles to the small, dense LDL particles of pattern B. The message here is that not only is a standard low-fat, moderate-to-high carbohydrate diet not appropriate for everyone but that, beyond matching nutrition therapy to genotype in order to maximize effectiveness of therapy, mismatching the two may actually cause harm. Similarly, Superko and colleagues have found that drug therapy needs to be matched to the LDL particle pattern type as well (Superko et al., 1997).

Another genetic locus that is being investigated as a predictor of cardiovascular risk is the apolipoprotein E (apo E) gene (*APOE*). Variation in this gene is associated with differences in the risk of both developing premature atherosclerosis and developing Alzheimer's disease. The normal allele (variant) is the *E3* allele, and most people are homozygous for *E3/E3*. Abnormal variants are the *E2* and *E4* alleles. Varying study designs make it difficult to define the effect of each allele clearly, but, in general, those with *E4/E4* or *E4/E3* have increased total cholesterol and LDL-C levels compared with those homozygous for the normal alleles (*E3/E3*). Those with at least one *E2* allele tend to have lower total cholesterol and LDL-C levels than those with an *E3* or *E4* allele. As with LDL particle density, attempts are being made to correlate *APOE* genotype with cardiovascular risk susceptibility, pharmacologic treatment, and diet and exercise treatment in order to define the most effective therapy associated with each genotype.

The situation with apo E is further complicated in that the pattern varies with age, which suggests that the effect of genetic variation in the *APOE* gene on plasma lipids can be modified and that age is one such modifying factor. Sex is another modifying factor, with a response in plasma lipid concentrations seen in men more than in women. The influence of *APOE* variant with alcohol intake is also clouded by the sex factor: men with the *E4* allele who drink alcohol have higher plasma LDL-C levels, but women with the *E4* allele have higher LDL-C levels irrespective of alcohol status (Corella et al., 2001). Not surprisingly, given the varying study designs and the potential for external factors to modify genetic outcomes, there are inconsistent data at present.

In terms of dietary approaches, the *E4* allele appears to be most responsive to dietary fat manipulation (Dreon et al., 1995). In contrast, the *E2* allele has poor plasma lipid responses to a low-fat diet but responds instead to exercise and reduced dietary carbohydrate and triglyceride (Erkkilä et al., 2001). In studying men and women with coronary artery disease, those with the *E2* allele had lower LDL-cholesterol levels than did those with the other variants, but they had higher triglyceride levels. The allele was found to be associated with elevated triglyceride levels related to dietary sucrose ingestion. Implications for nutrition professionals include developing dietary approaches that minimize simple carbohydrate intake for those homozygous or heterozygous for the *E2* allele and focusing on dietary fat modification for those with an *E3* or *E4* allele.

A newly discovered gene, *APOA-V*, has been located on chromosome 11 close to the apolipoprotein gene cluster that contains the genes for apolipoproteins A-I, C-III, and A-IV. Apo A-V is thought to influence triglyceride levels in humans (Pennacchio et al., 2001). Transgenic mice that overexpressed the gene had triglyceride levels at one-third those of the controls; *APOA-V* knockout mice had levels four times higher than the controls. The gene is polymorphic, and it may be possible to use polymorphisms to predict who is susceptible to elevated triglyceride levels and then to target low-carbohydrate diets to this population. Interestingly, this gene was first found in mice; by using the extensive databases now available as a result of the Human Genome Project, the comparable gene was located in humans and subsequently studied. At least three SNPs have been detected that correlate with elevated triglyceride levels and can potentially be used as markers to screen populations for those at risk, who could then be counseled on ways to minimize expression of this disorder.

Hypertension

Hypertension is also a multigenic/multifactorial disorder. It takes several genes and several environmental factors for most people to develop hypertension. Risk increases with age, is greater in men than in women, and in African Americans than in Caucasians. A variety of factors is involved; sodium is just one factor and affects blood pressure in only a portion of hypertensive individuals. As the gene-protein-nutrient associations sort out, nutrition professionals will need to reconsider hypertensive therapy in relation to sodium restriction.

Type 2 Diabetes Mellitus

Type 2 diabetes is another example of a genetically complex chronic disorder that is being studied using a genetic approach. As with cardiovascular disease, there are multiple genes controlling the various aspects of blood sugar regulation, from the regulation of insulin production to the cascade of events involved in translocating glucose into the cell. Some 150 different genotypes, including mitochondrial mutations, have been associated with the phenotype of glucose intolerance that characterizes type 2 diabetes (Berdanier, 2001).

Newly discovered genes associated with the development of type 2 diabetes, even though not carried by the majority of people, can be helpful in studying gene-disease associations and the influence of nutrition and other environmental factors. The Oji-Cree aboriginal people in northern Ontario are an isolated population with a high incidence of obesity-related type 2 diabetes when these individuals consume diets high in sugar and saturated fat (Hegele et al., 2000; Hegele 2001a, b). Diabetes was virtually unreported in this population just fifty years ago, which makes it an interesting population for studying environmental influences on gene expression. Changes in lifestyle practices have been accompanied by expression of genetic information that was previously silent in terms of clinical manifestations.

One of the outcomes of the studies with the Oji-Cree population has been the identification of an allele, the G319S mutation in the *HNF1A* (hepatocyte nuclear factor-1) gene, that is unique to this population. The immediate application to practice is limited, since most nutrition professionals do not routinely see clients from this population, but the finding of a unique mutation that's directly associated with type 2 diabetes is helpful in sorting out the details of the molecular basis for type 2 diabetes. Once such mutations surface within a population, they provide the basis for a diagnostic test for disease susceptibility. Depending on how widespread the mutation is among other populations, the diagnostic test may be broadly applicable for screening or confined to a particular population. The economics of diagnostic testing aside, once diagnosed, medical and nutritional interventions can be implemented.

Another diabetes-associated mutation has been identified in Europeans from the Botnia region of Finland; in the Mexican-American population of Starr County, Texas; and in the Pima Indians of Arizona, who have the highest known incidence of type 2 diabetes in the world (Horikawa et al., 2000). The gene, *CAPN10*, is a member of the calpain-like cysteine protease family and codes for the protein calpain-10, a metabolic pathway never before associated with diabetes. The relevance here is that such a finding puts us one step closer to a diagnostic test that can detect diabetes susceptibility early in a person's life. When the details of the gene's effect on the development of diabetes are available, we may discover novel nutritional approaches to either preventing or ameliorating type 2 diabetes associated with this mutation.

An interesting aspect of diabetes in terms of the importance of associating nutrition therapy with the genetic basis for a disorder is the finding that over forty mutations in the DNA of the mitochondrial genome result in the phenotype of diabetes mellitus (Berdanier, 2001). Nutrition therapy for diabetes resulting from mitochondrial mutations needs to be distinct from that for diabetes resulting from nuclear (chromosomal) mutations. Mitochondrial diabetes is not typical type 2 diabetes. Weight loss is not a normal part of therapy because these individuals tend to be of normal weight. Exercise is usually not a cornerstone of therapy because in many of these individuals the mutation affects ATP production in skeletal muscle. In fact, many accumulate lactate because of impaired pyruvate utilization. The significance to nutrition professionals is that the mutation has a primary bearing on biochemistry and physiology and thus on both medical and nutrition therapy. The present tendency in diabetes diagnostics is to conclude that if an individual does not have type 1 diabetes, the individual almost certainly has type 2 diabetes. Treating a person with mitochondrial-based diabetes with conventional type 2 therapy would be a mistake. At a minimum, such treatment would not have the desired positive outcome; at a maximum, it may be downright harmful to the client. Further, clinicians tend to overlook the possibility of mitochondrial-based diabetes. A genetics-savvy nutrition professional who is alert to this possibility can help both the physician and the client maximize therapeutic outcomes.

Type 2 diabetes is characterized by insulin resistance and premature atherosclerosis, an interrelationship that is puzzling to many. Genetic studies are helping to dissect this complex interrelationship, with the expectation that insight will be gained into the fundamental mechanisms of disease that will, in turn, lead to useful therapeutic approaches. The autosomal dominant Dunnigan-type familial partial lipodystrophy (FPLD) is strikingly similar to the metabolic syndrome (Syndrome X) that often precedes the development of overt type 2 diabetes: central obesity, hyperinsulinemia, hyperlipidemia (LDL-C and triglycerides), hypertension, low levels of HDL-C, and early-onset cardiovascular disease. Mutations that give rise to FPLD do not, however, code for proteins that would be expected to be involved in the pathogenesis of type 2 diabetes nor of cardiovascular disease (Hegele, 2001c). They code for proteins that form the nuclear envelope that protects the contents of the cell nucleus. The gene is polymorphic, so variants and their effects on insulin resistance and atherosclerosis can be studied. These types of mutations help expand the inquiry into how these two conditions may be interrelated. Through the use of animal models and manipulation of the genes and their environmental signals, what is now a confusing muddle will, ultimately, sort out into useful therapeutic approaches. Although not immediately applicable clinically, the fact that additional genes are being discovered that give rise to the phenotype of diabetes mellitus should alert clinicians to the need to keep an open mind as to what constitutes "standard" therapy for type 2 diabetes, a disease whose prevalence is escalating.

Other Chronic Disorders

Additionally, chronic disorders such as the inflammatory bowel disorders, obesity, and osteoporosis are being studied in terms of their underlying genetic bases and the impact of various alleles on dietary response. Recently a major gene in the development of Crohn's disease was discovered, which has helped to distinguish this inflammatory bowel disorder from ulcerative colitis (Rioux et al., 2001). As the gene's role in inflammation and response to anti-inflammatory nutrients and dietary supplements becomes clear, it may be possible to target nutrition therapy to Crohn's disease beyond just the use of anti-inflammatory agents such as curcumin and omega-3 fatty acids.

Obesity is another complex disorder that is likely a catch-all category for several different disorders, each determined by different genes and responsive to different environmental signals, but all manifesting as obesity. Here twin studies have been helpful in establishing that genetics sets the base but environmental factors play a major role in determining who among the susceptible will become obese. What is needed are good animal models in which the various aspects of obesity can be isolated and combined under controlled circumstances. The transgenic mouse, once again, appears to be a promising system for genetic-based obesity research.

With osteoporosis, the vitamin D receptor is a key player in building and maintaining adequate bone mineral density. The gene that codes for the receptor (VDR) is polymorphic, and there appears to be an association between the genotype and hip and spine bone mineral density in adults. Specific variants at this locus have been found to influence bone mineral density response to calcium and to caffeine intake (Rapuri, 2001). Similarly, a mutation in an unidentified gene has been found to lead to exceptionally dense bone mineralization. Knowing the genotype of such individuals is essential to tailoring dietary approaches to the biochemistry of the individual. In a woman with the VDR variant that causes an increased rate of bone loss in response to caffeine, attention would be given to limiting caffeine intake, whereas this approach may not be needed in a woman with the normal variant. Calcium recommendations would vary depending upon whether the woman had a VDR variant that absorbed calcium poorly or had the gene that leads to greater than normal bone mineralization, in which case excess calcium might be deposited in the soft tissues and be harmful to her.

Obviously, genotype will determine the direction of therapy, whether medical, pharmacological, or nutritional. Ultimately, the details of exactly how the key nutrients for each of these disorders influences genetic outcomes will become available and will serve as the basis for developing therapeutic approaches.

GENETICS AND DIETARY SUPPLEMENTS

The same foundation that underlies pharmacogenomics is important in considering the ability of individuals to use dietary supplements safely and effectively, particularly herbal supplements. These supplements appear to be metabolized by the same detoxification enzymes of the gut and liver that metabolize medications. The polymorphisms in the cytochrome P450 enzymes, particularly in the primary drug-metabolizing enzyme, intestinal CYP 3A4, are expected to affect herbal supplement metabolism in the same way they affect the metabolism of drugs and other xenobiotics (compounds not normally found in the body). The recent findings that components of the herb St. John's wort strongly induce CYP 3A4 and thereby alter the metabolism of drugs taken along with St. John's wort have launched a number of studies dedicated to investigating the metabolism of some of the more popular herbal supplements (Moore et al., 2000; Wentworth et al., 2000).

Like herbs, foods have their own mix of botanical compounds, xenobiotics, and carcinogens from both plant and animal sources and should also be considered from the standpoint of the match between the components in food and the genetic makeup of the individual. Components in grapefruit juice, for example, inhibit this same cytochrome P450 enzyme that St. John's wort induces (Lown et al., 1997). Although by different mechanisms, both types of botanical components interfere with the metabolism of certain oral medications and alter the therapeutic efficacy of those drugs.

Virtually any food or dietary supplement requires metabolic enzymes and transport proteins to convert it into products that are useful to cells. Depending on the genetic makeup of the individual, the conversion of these substances will vary. Ultimately, the goal is to match nutrients, whether from food or dietary supplements, to the individual's genetic makeup. Unfortunately, our knowledge is too limited at this point to be able to do such matching beyond a superficial level, but this approach is the future direction for nutritional genomics and will ultimately be reached.

PRACTICAL APPLICATIONS: USING NUTRITION TO MODIFY GENETIC OUTCOMES

As nutrition therapy shifts toward a gene-based approach, nutrients will be used as therapeutic agents to improve faulty biochemistry caused by genetic mutations. This shift has already begun, but we can expect it to gain momentum as the mechanisms of disease are unraveled and the specifics of nutrient-gene associations are discovered. As genetic profiling becomes more sophisticated, nutrition counseling will involve the development of nutrition therapy tailored to a patient's genotype. What does this look like in practice?

Taking a Thorough Family History

The first step is to take, and use, a thorough family history. One of the wonderful advantages of being a nutrition professional is that we often have more time with the patient/client than other members of the patient's health care team do. Identifying and factoring in individual genetic variations and personal preferences is time-consuming, and the nutrition professional makes a valuable contribution to the care of the patient in this regard.

Include a thorough family history in your comprehensive assessment. At minimum, gather the following information about all first-degree relatives (parents, siblings, offspring) and, preferably, three generations of family members:

- The gender of each family member
- The relationships among all family members and whether these are biologically related
- The age of each family member and the age at death, if appropriate (the information is conventionally recorded from oldest to youngest)
- All miscarriages and stillbirths or other pregnancy complications
- All adoptions
- The diseases associated with each family member
- The presence of consanguinity, if it exists
- The ethnic background of the family
- The date the pedigree was drawn
- The name of the person who provided the data
- A plan for keeping the family history updated with new births, deaths, and disease diagnoses

Record this information in standard pedigree format, and file it in the medical record. Many practitioners take a family history but record it in narrative form. Statements like "Mary's grandfather and two of her aunts died of colon cancer" are common but not informative. Was it Mary's maternal grandfather or paternal grandfather? Were her aunts her father's sisters, her mother's sisters, or one of each? Are they biologically related to Mary's grandfather who had colon cancer? These relationships are important in assessing Mary's need for genetic counseling. A pedigree clarifies relationships and disease associations in ways that the narrative format does not. Basic pedigree notation can be found in most medical genetics textbooks. By convention, paternal information is recorded on the left side of the pedigree and maternal information on the right. Children and siblings are listed in order of age, from oldest to youngest. Be sure to keep the generations separate, with grandparents of the patient on the top line; the patient's parents on the second line; the patient and the patient's siblings and first cousins on the third line; and the patient's children, nieces, and nephews on the fourth line. Each generation is numbered with a roman numeral beginning with I for the grandparents on down. The individuals in each generation are then numbered 1, 2, 3, and so on from left to right. See a medical genetics text such as that by Jorde and colleagues, listed under Useful Resources.

Before you begin collecting family history data, discuss what you are doing with your client and how the information will be used. The questions are quite personal and may bring up sensitive family issues. Plus, many people do not know their genetic history, and unearthing the information can take time and provoke aggravation that they will be more willing to endure if they understand how the information will be useful.

When analyzing the family history, look for those disorders that you know to be more common than may be typically appreciated, because they are often overlooked by others. Early detection is another valuable contribution that the nutrition member of the health care team can make. For example, the gluten-sensitive enteropathies and the iron-overload disorder hemochromatosis, discussed earlier, are common and frequently not detected early in the course of the disease. These appear to be recessive disorders inherited in a straightforward Mendelian fashion, which allows you to predict who is homozygous and who is heterozygous. Armed with this information, you and the physician can map out a strategy for medical surveillance or early intervention for your client and other family members using a combination of medical and nutritional therapies.

One of the concepts that is changing is our thinking that the carrier individual, the heterozygote, is functionally normal and does not need medical or nutritional attention. Particularly with autosomal recessive disorders, the assumption is that individuals are "normal" unless they have two genes containing the mutation responsible for the disorder. However, in the monogenic disorder familial hypercholesterolemia, there is variability among carriers in response to environmental factors, which can modulate the severity of the disease (Hegele, 2002). In the case of gluten-sensitive enteropathy, or hemochromatosis (where transport of a toxic mineral is elevated), what happens in the heterozygote when the faulty protein is present at 50 percent of the level seen in the toxic state but also at 50 percent higher than the level seen in the normal individual? Very likely these individuals will have at least some degree of impairment. A thought for nutrition professionals to consider is that, given the high incidence of these latter two disorders in the Caucasian population (homozygous: 1 in 250 to 500 individuals; heterozygous: 1 in 8 to 10) and the strong dependency on an iron-enriched, wheat-based diet in this country, there is likely a much higher incidence of latent disease than is appreciated. Early identification of carrier individuals and appropriate testing may identify an impairment that can be addressed before the full-blown disorder develops.

Also, be alert to disorders in the pedigree where the primary lesion is not thought to be nutritional. For example, the single-gene disorder cystic fibrosis (CF) is common among Caucasians. It is inherited as an autosomal recessive and, until recently, has not been thought to be related directly to nutrition. The disease results from a defect in the gene coding for a membrane protein involved in the transport of sodium and chloride across the epithelia of the lung and intestinal mucosa. Those with the disease experience mucus buildup in the lungs and often suffer from chronic lung inflammation and frequent respiratory infections that result. Pancreatic insufficiency is also a common complication. Recent work with a mouse model that mimics cystic fibrosis found that these mice had abnormally high levels of the omega-6 fatty acid arachidonic acid (AA) and abnormally low levels of the omega-3 fatty acid docosahexaenoic acid (DHA) in those organs most affected by CF: lungs, pancreas, and intestines (Freedman et al., 1999). Feeding DHA to these mice for one week corrected the imbalance and also reversed the signs of CF. If this promising finding holds true for humans, nutrition professionals will be called on to assist CF patients and their families in increasing their dietary intake of DHA while decreasing intake of arachidonic acid. Further, this approach is likely to work with some of the 1,000 variants that have been described for the CF gene, but not for others. Genetics-savvy nutrition professionals who are familiar with the underlying genetic variation will understand the basis for the variability in dietary response. Ultimately, the DNA sequence of each individual's genotype will be available, and there will be no need to guess which variant will respond to which dietary approach.

Becoming the Genetics Point Person on the Health Care Team

It's certainly within the physician's scope of practice to test, diagnose, and discuss the implications with clients and their families. The genetics-savvy nutrition professional, however, can be a major asset in helping the physician in understanding the genetics of the condition and the potential for nutritional intervention and in translating the disease and the chosen therapies to the client. Given the time constraints of today's practice, it's often the nutrition professional who answers many of the client's questions, directs the client to reliable resources for further education, and identifies effective support resources.

Some specific suggestions follow for ways to enhance the health care team's effectiveness as it develops expertise in incorporating genetics into practice:

- With children, use a normal physical exam to watch for failure to thrive and little or no response with diet therapy.
- Also watch for recurrent infections; metabolic disorders often result in immune dysfunction, and the child is susceptible to infections.
- Be alert for similar problems in other siblings.
- Liver dysfunction is common to many disorders of metabolism; persistent elevation of hepatic enzymes is a red flag at any age.
- In adults, watch for gluten intolerance and hemochromatosis.

Becoming Knowledgeable about Frequently Encountered Diseases

For those diseases that are of particular interest to you, either personally or by virtue of your practice setting, become an expert in the underlying genetic and biochemical bases. This process is time consuming and never ending as genetic research barrels forward at a dizzying pace. Know the well documented uses of food and dietary supplements for these conditions, and know how to use food and supplements to address genetic limitations. Use your background knowledge and clinical experience to develop logical, science-based approaches that will not harm the client and stand an excellent chance of helping him or her.

Obviously, all the knowledge and skills we've acquired to date are needed: biochemistry and nutrition, which foods are good sources of the nutrients needed and in what amounts, which dietary supplements can be helpful and in which dosages, and how to recognize quality. Above all, keep an open mind. Therapies are going to change dramatically. We will be moving away from the simplistic, one-size-fits-all approach and toward the nutrition-by-design approach.

Getting Started on the Journey

The sheer magnitude of what we need to know can be overwhelming. It helps to remember that nutrition professionals already have an excellent base upon which to build. Some of it may be rusty, but it's still there. Begin by developing a background in basic genetics and the genetics-nutrition connection. In particular, focus on learning the terminology; the connections among genes, disease, and nutrition; how diseases arise and how they're inherited at the chromosomal, mitochondrial, or molecular level; how nutrition ties in with genetics in terms of health and disease (this area will be ever changing over the next couple of decades); the many contributions that nutrition professionals can make in this area; and where to find useful information.

Identify an area that you're particularly interested in, which may be the focus of your professional work, or a health condition that you or a loved one has. Become an expert on its biochemical basis and learn what is known about the genetics of that disorder. Learn how the disease is inherited and how it's detected. Can the carrier be detected? Is the carrier functionally impaired? Is there anything you can do nutritionally to improve the functioning of the homozygote or heterozygote? Investigate the ethnic groups in which the disease is most prevalent, if any; for example, celiac disease is particularly prevalent in those of Irish descent, whereas adenomatous polyposis colon cancer is increased in frequency among Ashkenazi (eastern European) Jews, who are also at high risk for Tay-Sachs disease. Work together with the physician to educate yourself about the red flags to watch for in the client and in the medical record and learn what can be done medically and nutritionally once these red flags are detected.

Build an integrated team in which the members cover one another's backs, so that together you're likely to cover all the bases in this emerging area of applying genetics to clinical practice. This can only improve the health care of the client and increase your value to the team. Develop your own personal continuing education program:

■ Read journals pertinent to your focus area. The *Journal of the American Medical Association* and the *New England Journal of Medicine* regularly carry articles that discuss genetics and health. *Nature Medicine* adds more depth on the genetics end. *Scientific American* and the *New York Times* do a great job of providing the big picture for a topic and of translating complex concepts into everyday language. Sometimes having a simplified overview as an introduction to a new topic is helpful in developing a framework to which you can add details over time.

■ Attend meetings in your focus area. Increasingly, subject area meetings are including genetics as it becomes obvious that genetics is central to disorders within that focus. The annual joint meetings of the American Society of Medical Genetics and the March of Dimes are good sources for background information and clinical applications of genetics. Ultimately nutrition conferences will be incorporating genetics regularly.

■ Network. Network with nutrition professionals, physicians, nurses, and pharmacists who incorporate genetics into their practices. Network with genetics counselors and physicians and with Ph.D.s who have specialty training in clinical genetics.

Nutrition therapy can play many roles in improving genetic outcomes. Single-gene disorders with clear-cut gene/disease/nutrient modulation effects will likely be the first practical applications of this approach. The chronic disorders, which appear to involve complex interactions of multiple genes and multiple environmental factors, will require considerably more research to become amenable to gene-directed nutrition therapy. Genes determine a wide variety of protein-based components in the cell: enzymes, receptors, cofactors, structural components, lipoproteins, hormones and other mediators, and structural components such as those that determine blood clotting and blood pressure. Most of the known genes for these proteins are polymorphic. It will be interesting to track which of these genes and their products respond to nutritional modulation and to learn how to influence genetic outcomes.

Useful Resources

Ames BN, Elson-Schwab I, Silver EA. High-dose vitamin therapy stimulates variant enzymes with decreased coenzyme binding affinity (increased K(m)): relevance to genetic disease and polymorphisms. *Am J Clin Nutr.* 2002; 75:616–658.

Austin MA, King MC, Vranizan KM, Krauss RM. Atherogenic lipoprotein pheno-type: a proposed genetic marker for coronary heart disease risk. *Circulation.* 1990; 82:495–506.

Benoit P, Emmanuel F, Caillaud JM, et al. Somatic gene transfer of human apo A-I inhibits atherosclerosis progression in mouse models. *Circulation.* 1999; 99:105–110.

Berdanier CD. Nutrient-gene interactions. *Nutr Today.* 2000; 35:8–17.

Berdanier CD. Mitochondrial gene expression in diabetes mellitus: effect of nutrition. *Nutr Rev.* 2001; 59:61–70.

Bertram JS. Carotenoids and gene regulation. *Nutr Rev.* 1999; 57:182–191.

Blanchard RK, Cousins RJ. Regulation of intestinal gene expression by dietary zinc: induction of uroguanylin mRNA by zinc deficiency. *J Nutr.* 2000; 130:1393S–1398S.

Blanchard RK, Moore JB, Green CL, Cousins RJ. Inaugural article: modulation of intestinal gene expression by dietary zinc status: effectiveness of cDNA arrays for expression profiling of a single nutrient deficiency. *Proc Natl Acad Sci USA.* 2001; 98:13507–13513.

Busch CP, Hegele RA. Genetic determinants of type 2 diabetes mellitus. *Clin Genet.* 2001; 60:243–254.

Cao SX, Dhahbi JM, Mote PL, Spindler SR. Genomic profiling of short- and long-term caloric restriction effects in the liver of aging mice. *Proc Natl Acad Sci USA.* 2001; 98:10630–10635.

Clarke SD. Nutrient regulation of gene and protein expression. *Curr Opin Clin Nutr Metab Care.* 1999; 2:287–289.

Clarke SD. Polyunsaturated fatty acid regulation of gene transcription: a molecular mechanism to improve the metabolic syndrome. *J Nutr.* 2001; 131:1129–1132.

Clarke SD, Thuillier P, Baillie RA, Sha X. Peroxisome proliferator-activated receptors: a family of lipid-activated transcription factors. *Am J Clin Nutr.* 1999; 70:566–571.

Corella D, Tucker K, Lahoz C, et al. Alcohol drinking determines the effect of the *APOE* locus on LDL-cholesterol concentrations in men: the Framingham Offspring Study. *Am J Clin Nutr.* 2001; 73:736–745.

Davis JN, Kucuk O, Sarkar FH. Genistein inhibits NF-kappa B activation in pros-tate cancer cells. *Nutr Cancer.* 1999; 35:167–174.

Desvergene B, Wahli W. Peroxisome proliferator-activated receptors: nuclear control of metabolism. *Endocr. Rev.* 1999; 20:649–688.

Dreon DM, Fernstrom HA, Miller B, Krauss RM. Low-density lipoprotein subclass patterns and lipoprotein response to a reduced-fat diet in men. *FASEB J.* 1994; 8:121–126.

Dreon DM, Fernstrom HA, Miller B, Krauss RM. Apolipoprotein E isoform phe-notype and LDL subclass response to a reduced-fat diet. *Arterioscler Thromb Vasc Biol.* 1995; 15:105–111.

Dreon DM, Fernstrom HA, Williams PT, Krauss RM. Reduced LDL particle size in children consuming a very-low-fat diet is related to parental LDL-subclass patterns. *Am J Clin Nutr.* 2000; 71:1611–1616.

Erkkilä AT, Sarkkinen ES, Lindi V, et al. APOE polymorphism and the hypertriglyceridemic effect of dietary sucrose. *Am J Clin Nutr.* 2001; 73:746–752.

Freedman SD, Katz MH, Parker EM, et al. A membrane lipid imbalance plays a role in the phenotypic expression of cystic fibrosis in cftr(-/-) mice. *Proc Natl Acad Sci USA.* 1999; 96:13995–14000.

Guengerich FP. Functional genomics and proteomics applied to the study of nutritional metabolism. *Nutr Rev.* 2001; 59:259–263.

Hegele RA. Genes and environment in type 2 diabetes and atherosclerosis in aboriginal Canadians. *Curr Atheroscler Rep.* 2001a; 3:216–221.

Hegele RA. Monogenic dyslipidemias: window on determinants of plasma lipoprotein metabolism. *Am J Hum Genet.* 2001b; 69:1161–1177.

Hegele RA. Premature atherosclerosis associated with monogenic insulin resistance. *Circulation.* 2001c; 103:2225–2229.

Hegele RA, Cao H, Hanley AJ, et al. Clinical utility of HNF1A genotyping for diabetes in aboriginal Canadians. *Diabetes Care.* 2000; 23:775–778.

Hegele RA, Huff MW, Young TK. Common genomic variation in LMNA modulates indexes of obesity in Inuit. *J Clin Endocrinol Metab.* 2001; 86:2747–2751.

Hines LM, Stampfer MJ, Ma J, et al. Genetic variation in alcohol dehydrogenase and the beneficial effect of moderate alcohol consumption on myocardial infarction. *N Engl J Med.* 2001; 344:549–555.

Horikawa Y, Oda N, Cox NJ, et al. Genetic variation in the gene encoding calpain-10 is associated with type 2 diabetes mellitus. *Nat Genet.* 2000; 26:163–175.

Jefferson LS, Kimball SR. Amino acid regulation of gene expression. *J Nutr.* 2001; 131:2460S–2466S.

Jorde LB, Carey JC, Bamshad MJ, White RL. *Medical Genetics.* St. Louis, Mo: Mosby, Inc.; 2000.

Jump DB, Clarke SD. Regulation of gene expression by dietary fat. *Annu Rev Nutr.* 1999; 19:63–90.

Kersten S, Desvergne B, Wahli W. Roles of PPARs in health and disease. *Nature.* 2000; 405:421–424.

Krauss RM. Heterogeneity of plasma low-density lipoproteins and atherosclerosis risk. *Curr Opin Lipidol.* 1994; 5:339–349.

Lamarche B, Tchernof A, Mauriege P, et al. Fasting insulin and apolipoprotein B levels and low-density lipoprotein particle size as risk factors for ischemic heart disease. *JAMA.* 1998; 279:1955–1961.

Lamarche B, Tchernof A, Moorjani S, et al. Small, dense low-density lipoprotein particles as a predictor of the risk of ischemic heart disease in men. Prospective results from the Quebec Cardiovascular Study. *Circulation.* 1997; 95:69–75.

Lown KS, Bailey DG, Fontana RJ, et al. Grapefruit juice increases felodipine oral availability in humans by decreasing intestinal CYP 3A protein expression. *J Clin Invest.* 1997; 99:2545–2553.

McCombs RJ, Marcadis DE, Ellis J, Weinberg RB. Attenuated hypercholesterolemic response to a high-cholesterol diet in subjects heterozygous for the apolipoprotein A-IV-2 allele. *N Engl J Med.* 1994; 331:706–710.

Moore LB, Goodwin B, Jones SA, et al. St. John's wort induces hepatic drug metabolism through activation of the pregnane X receptor. *Proc Natl Acad Sci USA.* 2000; 97:7500–7502.

Moustaïd-Moussa N, Berdanier C (eds). *Nutrient-Gene Interactions in Health and Disease.* Boca Raton, Fla: CRC Press; 2001.

Moya-Camarena SY, Belury MA. Species differences in the metabolism and regulation of gene expression by conjugated linoleic acid. *Nutr Rev.* 1999; 57:336–340.

Nagy L, Tontonoz P, Alvarez JG, et al. Oxidized LDL regulates macrophage gene expression through ligand activation of PPARgamma. *Cell.* 1998; 93:229–240.

Near SE, Wang J, Hegele RA. Single nucleotide polymorphisms of the very low-density lipoprotein receptor (VLDLR) gene. *J Hum Genet.* 2001; 46:490–493.

Nishini PM, Johnson JP, Naggert JK, Krauss RM. Linkage of atherogenic lipoprotein phenotype to the low-density lipoprotein receptor locus on the short arm of chromosome 19. *Proc Natl Acad Sci USA.* 1992; 89:708–712.

Palmer HJ, Paulson KE. Reactive oxygen species and antioxidants in signal transduction and gene expression. *Nutr Rev.* 1997; 55:353–361.

Pennacchio LA, Olivier M, Hubacek JA, et al. An apolipoprotein influencing triglycerides in humans and mice revealed by comparative sequencing. *Science.* 2001; 294:169–173.

Price PT, Nelson CM, Clarke SD. Omega-3 polyunsaturated fatty acid regulation of gene expression. *Curr Opin Lipidol.* 2000; 11:3–7.

Rapuri PB, Gallagher JC, Kinyamu HK, Ryschon KL. Caffeine intake increases the rate of bone loss in elderly women and interacts with vitamin D receptor genotypes. *Am J Clin Nutr.* 2001; 74:694–700.

Rioux JD, Daly MJ, Silverberg MS, et al. Genetic variation in the 5q31 cytokine gene cluster confers susceptibility to Crohn's disease. *Nat Genet.* 2001; 29:223–228.

Roberts MA, Mutch DM, German JB. Genomics: food and nutrition. *Curr Opin Biotechnol.* 2001; 12:516–522.

Sarkkinen E, Korhonen M, Erkkilä A, et al. Effect of apolipoprotein E polymorphism on serum lipid response to the separate modification of dietary fat and dietary cholesterol. *Am J Clin Nutr.* 1998; 68:1215–1222.

Schaefer EJ. Lipoproteins, nutrition, and heart disease. *Am J Clin Nutr.* 2002; 75:191–212.

Schaefer EJ, Heaton WH, Wetzel MG, Brewer HB Jr. Plasma apolipoprotein A-I absence associated with marked reduction of high density lipoproteins and premature coronary heart disease. *Arteriosclerosis.* 1982; 2:16–26.

Superko HR, Krauss RM, DiRicco C. Effect of HMGCoA reductase inhibitor (fluvastatin) on LDL peak particle diameter. *Am J Cardiol.* 1997; 80:78–81.

Teran-Garcia M, Rufo C, Nakamura MT, et al. NF-Y involvement in the polyunsaturated fat inhibition of fatty acid synthase gene transcription. *Biochem Biophys Res Commun.* 2002; 290:1295–1299.

Tontonoz P, Nagy L, Alvarez JG, et al. PPARgamma promotes monocyte/macrophage differentiation and uptake of oxidized LDL. *Cell.* 1998; 93:241–252.

Wentworth JM, Agostini M, Love J, et al. St John's wort, a herbal antidepressant, activates the steroid X receptor. *J Endocrinol.* 2000; 166:R11–16.

Xing N, Chen Y, Mitchell SH, Young CY. Quercetin inhibits the expression and function of the androgen receptor in LNCaP prostate cancer cells. *Carcinogenesis.* 2001; 22:409–414.

Xu J, Nakamura MT, Cho HP, Clarke SD. Sterol regulatory element binding protein-1 (SREBP-1) expression is suppressed by dietary polyunsaturated fatty acids: a mechanism for coordinate suppression of lipogenic genes by polyunsaturated fats. *J Biol Chem.* 1999; 274:23577–23583.

Xu J, Teran-Garcia M, Park JH, et al. Polyunsaturated fatty acids suppress hepatic sterol regulatory element-binding protein-1 expression by accelerating transcript decay. *J Biol Chem.* 2001; 276:9800–9807.

Useful Web Sites

There are not yet any sites dedicated to the use of gene-directed nutrition therapy. A limited number of educational sites that focus on genetics education for health care professionals are listed here.

The Foundation for Genetic Education & Counseling Web site. Available at: http://www.fgec.org/. Accessed August 1, 2002.

Human Genome Education Model Project Web site. Available at: http://www.georgetown.edu/research/gucdc/hugem/. Accessed August 1, 2002.

National Coalition for Health Care Professional Education in Genetics Web site. Available at: http://www.nchpeg.org/. Accessed August 1, 2002.

Additionally, numerous sites that offer genetics education or that pertain to the Human Genome Project can be found in the other chapters of this book.

7

Ethical, Legal, and Social Issues

The Human Genome Project is expected to have a profound ethical, legal, and social impact on our society. Ethical issues concern what is moral and right. Legal issues concern protections that the law should provide with regard to the use and ownership of information derived from genetic technologies. Social issues concern the effects of genetic advances on society and its members. The Human Genome Project has incorporated concerns about these ethical, legal, and social issues (often referred to collectively as *ELSI*) since its inception. In addition to ELSI concerns, there are economic concerns. Who should profit from the Human Genome Project? Each of these areas raises important questions.

In 1990, when the Human Genome Project began, an ELSI Program was established within both of the project's administrative arms: the National Human Genome Research Institute (NHGRI) of the U.S. National Institutes of Health (NIH), and the Office of Biological and Environmental Research (OBER) within the U.S. Department of Energy. The aim of both programs was to identify, analyze, and address the ELSI implications of the basic genetic research being conducted while this work was in progress. The ELSI programs have had the challenges of anticipating likely pressing issues and of funding, by means of grants, research and educational activities that address each of these issues. Attention is centered on four major areas:

- Privacy and fair use of genetic information
- Clinical integration of genetic technologies
- Ethical issues surrounding genetic research
- Professional education and resources

PRIVACY AND FAIRNESS IN THE USE AND INTERPRETATION OF GENETIC INFORMATION

ELSI-funded research into privacy and the fair use of genetic information is concerned with preventing discrimination or stigmatization by employers, insurers, or others based on an individual's genetic profile. The following list includes the types of activities and investigations supported to date:

- Assessing the effects of the Human Genome Project on access to medicines, health care, and insurance as well as the distribution of scarce medical resources
- Developing recommendations concerning these issues
- Analyzing the social and economic incentives and disincentives related to the use of various genetic testing and screening techniques
- Examining the issues surrounding genetic discrimination, genetic privacy legislation, and the attitudes of the insurance companies toward the use of genetic data
- Drafting a genetic privacy act
- Evaluating the effect of state and federal laws restricting health insurers' use of information that derives from genetic tests
- Working with organizations such as the U.S. Equal Employment Opportunity Commission (EEOC) and consumer groups such as the National Action Plan on Breast Cancer to strengthen consumer protection against workplace and health insurance discrimination

No specific federal genetic nondiscrimination legislation has been enacted to date, but some laws exist that provide a modicum of protection from genetic discrimination. The Americans with Disabilities Act of 1990 includes the protection of individuals with symptomatic genetic disorders to the same degree as those with any other disability. The Health Insurance Portability and Accountability Act of 1996 (HIPAA) directly addresses genetic discrimination by prohibiting the use of genetic information as a basis for denying coverage or even limiting eligibility for coverage. Genetic information in the absence of a diagnosis of illness cannot be considered a preexisting condition. An important limitation to HIPAA, however, is that it applies only to employer-based and commercially issued group health insurance. On February 8, 2000, President Bush signed an executive order prohibiting federal agencies from using genetic information in any hiring or promotion action. There are also HIPAA-related national standards now in place designed to ensure privacy of genetic information by limiting access to individuals' personal medication records.

The first steps have been taken to ensure privacy and fair use of genetic information, but many remain convinced that federal policy is required to protect against genetic discrimination in the workplace regarding individual insurance coverage.

CLINICAL INTEGRATION OF GENETIC TECHNOLOGIES

As new genetic technologies rapidly become available, many questions arise as to how best to integrate them into clinical practice. How reliable and useful is genetic testing? Are individuals properly prepared for testing and its outcomes? Should testing be carried out when there is no effective treatment for the disorder? ELSI-funded research in this area has focused on the following issues:

- Assessing the knowledge and attitude of the public concerning genetic testing and counseling
- Assessing the interest in and frequency of use of existing genetic testing
- Examining the impact that genetic technologies will have on individuals, families, and societies
- Assessing the psychosocial impact on individuals and families of having (or not having) genetic testing
- Evaluating the impact on health and illness of having information from genetic testing
- Determining the availability of and access to genetic testing
- Ensuring that genetic testing is performed by qualified laboratories with strict quality control programs in place
- Assessing the availability of adequately trained personnel to carry out and interpret the testing as well as to counsel the individuals and their families
- Reinforcing the need for appropriate informed consent procedures for individuals undergoing genetic testing
- Examining the financial aspects of genetic testing

To focus these broad-based efforts, the NHGRI established two research consortia targeted to cystic fibrosis (CF) and cancer, two diseases that are both common and of major societal concern. Within these focus areas, the consortia have developed recommendations for genetic testing, as well as clinical, laboratory, educational, and informed consent guidelines. For example, the consensus statement for cystic fibrosis recommends testing of all adults with a positive family history of CF, testing of partners of individuals with the disease, and offering testing to couples planning a pregnancy or seeking prenatal care. They do not, however, advocate screening of all newborns at this time. Recommendations were also made concerning the needs for continued research into CF, education about the disease, and genetic counseling services. The NIH Consensus Statement is available online (see Useful Web Resources section below).

Similar guidelines were developed and published in the *Journal of the American Medical Association* for breast, colon, and uterine cancer. Follow-up recommendations concerning the ELSI considerations of genetic testing for cancer were set forth in 1997 (Burke et al., 1997a and b; Geller et al., 1997).

A third initiative concerns genetic testing and accompanying guidelines for hereditary hemochromatosis (also called iron overload disease), a disorder that leads to the accumulation of excess iron in the body. The NHGRI collaborated with the Centers for Disease Control and Prevention in bringing together experts on this disorder to develop guidelines for the clinical and ELSI impact of identifying the gene(s) responsible for this disease (Burke et al., 1998). These recommendations formed the basis for a new research collaboration by the NHGRI and the National Heart, Blood, and Lung Institute to study relevant clinical and ELSI concerns. The possibility of population-wide screening for individual carriers of this disorder is also being addressed.

The next step for these initiatives is to broaden the focus to other diseases, particularly those associated with an aging population. A start has already been made in funding a study into the ELSI concerns relating to the introduction of testing for Alzheimer's disease and the potential for preventing or delaying Alzheimer's disease in high-risk population groups.

A number of other issues need to be addressed in this area, such as the availability of genetic services for specific populations; the impact of genetic research and technologies on societal systems such as families and communities; and the complex issues surrounding behavioral genetics, enhancement of an individual's genetic makeup, preimplantation genetic diagnosis, the ability to diagnose adult-onset disorders in children or even prenatally, and similar potential capabilities. The sophistication of the technologies that are becoming routine will greatly expand the options available and present ongoing challenges for staying on top of their ELSI implications.

ETHICAL ISSUES SURROUNDING GENETIC RESEARCH

The emphasis here is on the design of genetic research protocols and the informed consent process that accompanies such research studies. These studies include research involving pedigree analysis, gene discovery, genetic testing, gene therapy, large-scale genome sequencing, and genetic variation. Primary issues include the following:

- Ensuring the adequacy of informed consent on the part of participants in such studies to ensure that those entering into genetic research trials fully understand the potential risks and benefits of the treatment
- Protecting the privacy of participants related to the information and biological samples they provide for the research studies, including computer security
- Establishing restrictions, if any, that should be placed on genetic research with tissue samples that individuals have stored for possible future use
- Determining whether communities can exert significant peer pressure to force members to participate in such research studies, and if so, how to prevent such pressure to protect individual freedom of choice
- Awarding the rights to the intellectual property that results from research on biological samples donated by individuals

Some of the issues that remain to be addressed include the economic influence on genetic research and on the development of specific tests, the ethical influence on the design of genetic research, the cultural influences on research study design and execution, and the impact of the major focus on genetic research on the public perceptions of genetics.

PROFESSIONAL EDUCATION AND RESOURCES

The need to educate students, health care professionals, legal professionals, and other policy makers as well as the public on the ethical, legal, and social implications of genetic research has been a high priority of

ELSI-funded research since the inception of the Human Genome Project. Activities in this area include the following:

- Assessing the knowledge of health care professionals with regard to genetics and defining the needs for basic genetics education for this population
- Gathering information about the skill level of health care professionals with respect to their genetic testing recommendations, genetic counseling, and disorder-appropriate care
- Developing educational materials and seminars for health care professionals and consumers about genetics topics
- Educating legal professionals and policymakers with the goal of preparing the nation's courts to hear cases involving genetics and ELSI-related issues
- Educating high school and college students about genetics
- Developing university-level pilot courses on the implications of genetic research
- Broadcasting public service announcements concerning genetic science over public radio stations
- Providing resource materials to a wide-ranging audience through the Bioethicsline and GeneClinics online services; Bioethicsline provides online bibliographic information on bioethics literature, and GeneClinics provides bibliographic and practical medical genetics information (see "Useful Web Sites")

Those areas needing additional attention include determining what exactly each targeted population group needs to know about genetics, evaluating the extent to which the above activities have improved genetics literacy among such groups, and determining how various population groups best learn genetic concepts.

THOUGHTS TO PONDER

The new capabilities genetic technology is providing can be used to benefit or to harm society. Whether benefit or harm predominates is dependent on how intelligently we harness this powerful set of tools. Of particular concern to consumers and professionals alike are issues relating to genetic testing and therapy as well as the cloning of whole animals. Discussed here are just a few of the many questions that we as a society will need to address in the very near future.

Genetic Testing

Who should be tested? The ability to determine unequivocally that a patient carries the gene for a disorder for which there is an effective therapy is generally seen as beneficial. In time, there will likely be preventive steps that can be taken. Should we, however, test for a disorder for which there is no effective therapy? Should parents have the right to have their minor children tested? Can a person be required to be tested? After all, an individual who develops a debilitating disease represents a cost to society. Could that person be held responsible for failing to take preventive or therapeutic action known to prevent that disorder from developing?

Genetic testing is usually thought of in terms of testing for disease susceptibility, but it also includes testing for identification purposes. In both cases, DNA profiles would be stored in computerized databanks. It will likely become commonplace for an individual to be identified based on his genetic profile. Who should have access to such information? What should our policies be regarding information disclosure practices? Many people fear that such information will be used against them by life or health insurance companies or by employers. An employer who knows an employee is at increased risk of harm from toxic chemicals would be able to assign him or her to work in an area of the plant free of toxic chemicals. On the other hand, that employer might decline to hire that person in the first place in order to reduce the company's liability exposure. A child predisposed to disruptive behavior might receive early medical and psychological intervention. On the other hand, a school might discriminate against such a child. How will we protect against the misuse of genetic information?

Gene Therapy

Who should have access to gene-based therapy? Should there be an age limit? Should only those who can afford to pay have access? In whom should society make its gene therapy investment: in the bright young person with the promising future or the aging retiree? Should only those with life-threatening disorders have access? What about a person with albinism? Is this a necessary health procedure or a cosmetic one? Should parents-to-be have the right to enhance the inborn capabilities of their offspring through genetic therapy? Should insurance pay for this therapy? Who will decide? From which cells should the material for gene therapy come? Are fetal cells acceptable starting material from which to obtain the needed gene sequence? Is it acceptable to society for parents to conceive a child in order to provide cell transplants for a dying sibling?

Animal Cloning

Early successes in the cloning of animals have already been achieved, and cloned animals are already being used to produce milk containing medically valuable molecules. Society should begin to prepare itself for the day when cloning a human will be technically feasible. What would be the implications for society? In what ways might human cloning be beneficial or detrimental to society? Do we know enough to make these changes to the human genetic code wisely?

IMPLICATIONS FOR THE NUTRITION PROFESSIONAL

Clearly, there are more questions than answers at this point, but the Human Genome Project is spearheading debate in this area and pushing for the development of balanced approaches that will serve society well. Our responsibilities as citizens should be to anticipate the types of decisions that this new technology will require of us and to begin now to debate these issues in a considered way so that thoughtful policies can be developed.

As nutrition professionals, we will be involved in many of the ethical, legal, and social issues that our clients face. We can help to ensure that advances in genetics are used in ways that benefit our clients. Suggestions are offered here for each of the major issues.

Privacy and Fair Use of Genetic Information

Genetic information must be kept confidential, just as any other medical information is kept confidential. We as nutrition professionals should help our clients protect themselves against invasion of privacy by staying alert to the potential for abuse by others who may be in a position to obtain clients' genetic information. Nutrition professionals can also become actively involved in the development of state and federal legislation that will ensure genetic privacy and prevent discrimination.

Clinical Integration of Genetic Technologies

Nutrition professionals will be particularly helpful in the clinical integration of genetic technologies because nutrition and other lifestyle-related approaches will be the major therapeutic tools once a disorder (or susceptibility to one) has been detected by genetic testing. Many nutrition professionals are used to seeing a client after a physician has diagnosed a problem and has ordered a particular nutrition therapy for that client–a scenario that will change as genetic technologies are integrated into practice. Because genetics is a new addition to health care and few health care professionals are trained in genetic technologies or therapeutic options, good client care will require the entire health care team to work together to use these tools for the maximum benefit of the client. The nutrition professional will need to be familiar with the genetic testing process and the therapeutic options for the various test outcomes. Clients will want to discuss the whole situation with their various health care providers, and physicians will need the guidance that a knowledgeable nutrition professional can provide.

Ethical Issues Surrounding Genetic Research

Nutrition professionals involved in genetic research can play an important role in this team effort by helping to ensure that participants understand the seriousness of the matter and the potential outcomes of the experimental approach, and by providing valuable feedback to the other team members.

Professional Education and Resources

Educating ourselves, other health care professionals, and consumers of all ages about genetics, and particularly about the power of nutrition therapy, is another area in which nutrition professionals can have major impact. There is a place for all talents in the enormous task of developing a society that is knowledgeable about genetics. Beginning with our own client base, we can educate consumers about genetics and how nutrition can lessen disease susceptibility. Nutrition professionals with talents in writing, speaking, working with the media, or teaching classes will find any number of opportunities to educate generally about genetics and specifically about the ability of nutrition to modify gene expression.

Useful Resources

Burke W, Daly M, Garber J, et al. Recommendations for follow-up care of individuals with an inherited predisposition to cancer: II. BRCA1 and BRCA2. JAMA. 1997b; 277:997–1003.

Burke W, Petersen G, Lynch P, et al. Recommendations for follow-up care of individuals with an inherited predisposition to cancer: I. Hereditary nonpolyposis colon cancer. Cancer Genetics Consortium. *JAMA.* 1997a; 277: 915–919.

Burke W, Thomson E, Khoury MJ, et al. Hereditary hemochromatosis: gene discovery and its implications for population-based screening. *JAMA.* 1998; 280:172–178.

Geller G, Botkin JR, Green MJ, et al. Genetic testing for susceptibility to adult-onset cancer: the process and content of informed consent. *JAMA.* 1997; 277:1467–1474.

Wilfond B, Rothenberg K, Thomson E, Lerman C. Ethical and health policy issues in cancer genetic testing. *J Law Med Ethics.* 1997; 25:243–251.

Useful Web Sites

Baker C. Your Genes, Your Choices. Department of Energy Web site. Available at: http://www.ornl.gov/hgmis/publicat/genechoice/index.html. Accessed August 6, 2002. [Hard copies are available from AAAS, 202/326–6454; Fax: 202/371–9849.]

Bioethics resources on the Web. National Institutes of Health Web site. Available at: http://www.nih.gov/sigs/bioethics/outsidenih.html#genetics. Accessed August 6, 2002.

ELSI: Ethical, legal, and social implications of human genetics research. National Human Genome Research Institute Web site. Available at: http://www.nhgri.nih.gov/ELSI/. Accessed August 6, 2002.

ELSI Research Planning and Evaluation Group (ERPEG) Report. National Human Genome Research Institute Web site. Available at: http://www.nhgri.nih.gov/ELSI/erpeg_report.html. Accessed August 6, 2002.

Genetic testing for cystic fibrosis. *NIH Consens Statement* [serial online]. 1997;15(4):1–37. Available at: http://odp.od.nih.gov/consensus/cons/106/106_statement.htm. Accessed August 6, 2002.

Human Genome Project information: ethical, legal, and social issues. Department of Energy Web site. Available at: http://www.ornl.gov/hgmis/elsi/elsi.html. Accessed August 6, 2002.

Human Genome Project page. National Human Genome Research Institute Web site. Available at: http://www.nhgri.nih.gov. Accessed December 26, 2001.

Young EWD. The genetic revolution: Ethical issues. Access Excellence Web site. Available at: http://www.accessexcellence.org/AE/AEPC/BE02/gentest/gentoc.html. Accessed August 6, 2002.

8

Nutrition Policy

Advances in genetic research will dramatically change nutrition practice. Genotype profiling of individuals holds the promise of promoting health and increasing the *goodness of fit* between our genes and the foods we eat, thereby enhancing health and decreasing the risk of disease. The food supply will be affected as genetic capability expands and the demand grows for developing foods that can improve this goodness of fit. With each of these potentials comes risks, benefits, and issues that need to be considered from a policy perspective. In this chapter we will explore a number of these issues and their implications.

HEALTH PROMOTION–RELATED POLICY

Genetic research will have a dramatic impact on how we view health. Rather than viewing illness as something that happens to us, we will begin to see health as something we can make happen to ourselves. Medicine will change from disease-based to patient-based management. Nutrition will emerge as the central science of preventive medicine and will focus on matching diet to individual genotype, with the goal of alleviating existing disease and preventing future disease. Public health will begin to focus on maximizing genetic potential as a way to promote health and minimize disease. Because genetics is new to all of these applications, policy development must address a wide range of genetics-related issues. Some of the issues relating to nutrition that will likely be addressed early on are discussed here.

Nutrition Policy for Individuals

The central issue affecting nutrition policy is that genes underlie our potential for wellness and illness as well as determine our ability to use food to support health and minimize disease. Virtually all policy issues stem from this fundamental fact. Clearly, nutrition applications of the future must be based on genes. At the individual level, genotype will guide nutrition therapy. For populations, genetic differences must be taken into consideration when developing dietary guidelines, both at the national and international levels. Nutrition professionals will gain a set of powerful tools for changing health outcomes, which will open opportunities never before available in terms of the magnitude and significance of the nutrition professional to health care.

Individual genotypes, serving as a guide to nutrition therapy, will need to be readily available in the same way that height, weight, and blood pressure data are part of the general information used to direct the practitioner. Policy considerations here include ensuring that this information can only be used to benefit the individual and not to deny access to opportunities. These genotypic profiles will also provide new ways to categorize people. We will need to consider how to execute this categorization in positive, useful ways without stigmatizing our clients.

Most consumers have had little opportunity for formal education in genetic principles and genetic applications. Policymakers will need to consider how best to go about providing basic information about the relationship of genetics to health, disease, and nutrition, as well as how best to craft gene-based nutrition messages for a public with little background in genetics.

Nutrition Policy for Populations

At the population level, genetics is teaching us that there is no such thing as an average person, a realization with implications at all levels. The practitioner will be more appreciative of the genetic variability within a client population and consider this variability as the likely basis for ineffectiveness of therapy. Researchers will need to consider that the randomized control trial, the gold standard of clinical trials, is based on averages. Much of our dietary advice at the population level tends to be of a one-size-fits-all nature. Public health officials will need to grapple with how to develop dietary guidelines that meet the needs of individuals while delivering messages simple enough to be incorporated into today's busy lifestyles. Specifically, we need to address the goodness of fit of our food supply (discussed in the next section), use caution in extrapolating data from one population to another, redefine what we mean by optimum nutrient levels, and move away from one-size-fits-all messages.

Food fitness: a genetic perspective   Genetics is teaching us that genes underlie our ability to use food to support health and that these genes have evolved imperceptibly over the past millennium. Given the rapid evolution of our food supply, consideration must be given to how well our food fits our genes—that is, the goodness of fit of our food supply to our genetically determined ability to use that food effectively. Today's diet may not be the best fit for human beings. Our genetic constitution was selected under much simpler dietary conditions than those we encounter today. Our ancestors evolved on a diet of lean meat, fish, and seafood; fruits and vegetables with a low glycemic index; and nuts and seeds (Eaton and Konner, 1985; Cordain et al., 2001). This diet is thought to have been high in complex carbohydrates, fiber, and antioxidants from plant foods; low in saturated fat and omega-6 fatty acids and high in omega-3 fatty acids. During the forty thousand years since this hunter-gatherer period in our early development, our food supply has undergone tremendous change, but our genetic makeup has not. Our present diet is based on grains, particularly wheat. Yet wheat was introduced only ten thousand years ago. The spontaneous mutation rate for DNA is estimated at only one-half percent every million years. It is worth considering that the genes relating to our digestive, absorptive, and metabolic capacities are not too different, if at all, from those of our ancestors and may not be well adapted to a grain-based diet. Incorporating our understanding of genetics into our thinking on this issue will have wide-ranging effects on agricultural policy and on how we view the human diet and develop dietary guidelines.

Populations and gene pools   Our ability to digest, absorb, and use food depends ultimately on how well the proteins encoded in our genes function. Dietary recommendations must take this fundamental fact into account. There are subtle but important differences in this regard among individuals and in the gene pools that make up populations. The more geographically isolated that populations have been from each other as they evolved, the more different they are genetically, and the more likely they are to have evolved on somewhat different diets. Clearly, there are not only individual differences that must be considered when developing dietary guidelines, but also population differences that must be taken into account.

This basic fact does not mean that findings from one population cannot be extrapolated to another population, but it does mean that we must do so with caution. Think of a population as a model system. When a model system is used in the laboratory to ask questions with implications for human beings, the system is developed to come as close to the human situation as feasible so that the results will be directly applicable. However, the researcher is aware of important differences and limitations. The findings of the model system are therefore then tested in human beings. So it is with populations: findings from one population should be considered for application to other populations, but they should be applied judiciously and with respect for the different genetic constitutions of the two populations.

What is optimum?   Now that we realize genes set the upper and lower limits of an individual's personal health continuum and that genetic differences among individuals are significant, our concept of the optimum nutrient level is changing. Instead of trying to develop set levels, below which deficiency is likely and above which optimal health is likely, we will have to determine the minimum and maximum nutrient levels for each genotype.

This approach is daunting but not quite as overwhelming as it seems at first glance. Human beings have significant genetic differences that make us unique and that lead to variable responses to virtually any type of food, medication, or therapy imaginable, but we are enough alike as a species that a foundational message can be developed that will apply to everyone at some level.

Reformulation of nutrition messages   Genetics is pulling us strongly away from a one-size-fits-all approach. Hopefully we will be able to develop a set of foundational messages that serve as the core recommendations for health promotion. The challenge will be for the practitioner to customize these core messages to each individual, and for those in practice and at the public health level to educate clients about how to distinguish between core recommendations and the modifications that are specific to their genotypes.

Nutrition Policy for Nutrition Professionals

Policy consideration must also be given to the changing scope of practice of the nutrition professional. Nutrition therapy based on genotypic profiles is a powerful tool and promises to expand the capability of the nutrition professional significantly. Consideration will need to be given to how best to handle this expanding role in terms of scope of practice limitations in reference to the other members of the health care team. The era of genetics will enhance the value of the nutrition professional to health care immeasurably. Will we rewrite the nutrition professional's scope of practice accordingly?

Nutrition Policy and the Profession of Nutrition

Nutrition professionals do not routinely have a seat at the international policymaking table, but we should. Sound nutritional policy is an essential foundation for any human endeavor in any nation. The goal of each nation is essentially to maximize the genetic potential of its citizens so that they can be maximally productive and enjoy the highest possible quality of life. Imagine what the human race could accomplish if it maximized its health and brain power through appropriate nutrition and other lifestyle choices. The advances in genetic research and their clear connection to health will help to drive home the message that nutrition must be a major focus of global programs and that nutrition professionals must be included in these decision-making processes.

FOOD-RELATED POLICY

Among the primary goals of nutrition policy on a global scale is ensuring a sufficient quantity of food for all. At the very least, this means ensuring that this food is of a quality that meets minimum nutritional needs; the maximum goal is to promote health and prevent disease. Both conventional plant and animal breeding and the newer genetic engineering techniques of food biotechnology are available for increasing yield and for improving the nutritional composition of plant and animal foods.

Much of the focus of our food-related nutrition policy has been on producing and distributing food that can prevent diseases arising from nutritional deficiencies. Malnutrition is a global issue: in underdeveloped countries, it's a matter of inadequate amounts of health-promoting food; in developed countries, by contrast, it's a matter of an overabundance of health-robbing foods. These basic issues must be addressed before we can superimpose on them a higher goal of eating to maximize the genetic potential of individuals, populations, and nations. Ultimately, however, a shift will be made toward providing sufficient quantities of the appropriate foods to maximize the genetic potential of people worldwide.

Conventional breeding techniques have been used for centuries to change the food supply in order to increase yield and improve food's flavor, appearance, quality, and hardiness during the growing process. In general, people are comfortable with conventional breeding. These methods, however, are slow, labor intensive, and inefficient from a genetic perspective. The tools now available through biotechnology can significantly improve on each of these limitations of conventional breeding. People are not, however, as comfortable with these newer approaches to altering the food supply. Changing the food supply, whether by traditional methods or by modern technology, is risky business. Introducing new technology to any process is inherently accompanied by risk; biotechnology is no exception. Nutrition policymakers have the challenge of minimizing these risks while maximizing the benefits, all the while staying mindful of the potential concerns that citizens may have worldwide.

There is no doubt that genetic technology has the potential to change the food supply and is already doing so. Policy issues that must be addressed include whether or not such food is safe for long-term consumption, whether genetically modified foods pose a threat to our global ecology in the long run, and whether changing the food supply at such a rapid pace is good from the perspective of matching food to genes that have not changed appreciably in the last forty thousand years.

Safety, whether of the food itself or of the environment that harbors plants with transferred genes, is the primary issue here. Certainly the potential exists to develop foods that are allergenic and can cause potentially life-threatening reactions in the unsuspecting people who eat them (Nordlee, 1996; Taylor and Hefle, 2001). The transferred genes code for proteins, and proteins can be allergenic. What must be evaluated is the likelihood that these allergenic proteins will be transferred into food crops. Certainly they can be, but will they be? What safeguards can be put in place to ensure that they are not? What is a reasonable test of safety that ensures a food is nonallergenic? Who regulates such activities?

Presently three agencies oversee the safety of our food supply: the United States Department of Agriculture (USDA), the Environmental Protection Agency (EPA), and the Food and Drug Administration (FDA). The USDA, through its Animal and Plant Health Inspection Service (APHIS), oversees the field-testing of plants developed using biotechnology. The EPA evaluates the pest-resistant properties of the plants. The FDA is charged with assessing the safety of all foods and animal feeds, irrespective of the technology used to develop them. At least one, and sometimes all three, of these agencies is involved in the regulatory process for foods produced through biotechnology.

This review process is considered sufficient by these U.S. governmental agencies and by the scientists who advise them. Recently, however, the public has become concerned about safety issues and has requested a mandatory premarket evaluation as well as a more transparent process by which the review is conducted and approval is granted. The FDA has responded to this public feedback and moved forward to provide premarket evaluation, to implement a more open review process, and to issue guidelines for manufacturers wishing to label their foods as having been developed or not developed using modern biotechnology methods.

Consumers with concerns about the safety of foods are requesting mandatory labeling; for the most part, the government and scientific communities feel such labeling is not warranted. The government's position is that the underlying technology has undergone significant scrutiny by the country's top scientific advisers for over thirty years and has been judged safe. In its opinion, the regulatory review now in place is sufficient to guard against potential harm. Voluntary labeling is presently an option. Mandatory labeling would require that foods produced using biotechnology be kept separate, from seed to market, from foods produced using conventional genetic methods, which would be challenging. This issue remains a contentious one, but it must be resolved.

Is the current activity by these three agencies sufficient to protect the consumer from the introduction of potentially harmful foods? Perhaps. No one can guarantee that eating any food for a lifetime will not have unforeseen negative consequences, particularly given the fact that each individual is genetically unique. However, whichever safeguards the government puts into place need to function appropriately. In a recent incident involving the Starlink variety of genetically engineered corn, the ability of the government to safeguard the food supply was called into question. Dual approval was granted for this strain of corn—it was approved for animal feed but not immediately approved for human consumption, because it contained a protein that is very slowly digested in the gut, a condition often seen with proteins that provoke allergic responses. The strain was subsequently approved for human use, but by that time, it had already entered the food supply. This incident points out two issues worth considering by policymakers: that it's relatively easy for unapproved foods to enter the human food supply, and that food ultimately intended for human consumption should not be released for animal consumption before it has been approved for human consumption as well.

EDUCATION-RELATED POLICY

The genetic revolution promises to have a significant impact on virtually all societies. In order to maximize this potential, members of a given society must be knowledgeable of the revolution taking place around them and its potential benefits. As alluded to earlier, neither consumers nor nutrition professionals are well versed in genetics at this time, a situation that needs to be addressed. Ideally, consumer education should begin in the elementary years. Genetics, its connection to health and disease, and the power of nutrition to maximize health and minimize disease should be incorporated into teachings about biology and health for all ages. Dissemination of information can take place through schools, churches and other community groups, governmental agencies, and, increasingly, through the Internet. We can start now with a focus on the link between genetics and health, and be ready to expand that message to genotype profiling as the drug-metabolizing–enzyme diagnostic tests become available. Nutrition should be included from the beginning and portrayed as a powerful tool for addressing the susceptibilities our genotypes will represent. Even at this early stage in our understanding of how to use nutrition in this way, we can begin to educate consumers about the responsibilities they will face as these tools become available, and the valuable role that the nutrition professional will assume in helping them weigh their options and decide a course of action.

Those in positions to guide the educational foundation of nutrition professionals should similarly begin to look for ways to introduce genetics into the curriculum of nutrition students and to provide opportunities for postgraduates. Chapter 9 gives several suggestions for what that foundation should include. It's a fast-changing environment for nutrition professionals today. The tremendous consumer interest in complementary therapies and dietary supplementation, coupled with the genetics revolution, is expanding the opportunities for nutrition professionals significantly and rapidly. Now would seem a good time to consider the future roles that nutrition professionals will play and to reorient the educational foundation accordingly. As the magnitude of training needs increases, we will have to be creative in how we pack all that information into a few short years at the university.

More than likely, we will not be able to pack it all in, and we will need to reframe education as a lifelong process that spans the entire career of the nutrition professional, beginning with college and easily continuing for many more decades. Rather than view the college years as the period in which one is educated, college may come to be viewed as a unique incubation period, during which the nutrition professional is taught how to self-educate. College years then become the time to learn and make mistakes under the tutelage of a more experienced professional. Once the student leaves the nest, how can we ensure that the education process remains dynamic and ever current for the postgraduate nutrition professional? Clearly, there is much work ahead, but the rewards of developing practitioners who make significant contributions to the global health more than match the challenge.

The future has never looked brighter for nutrition professionals. We are about to possess a powerful set of tools for maximizing genetic potential, which includes robust health and a level of quality of life never before experienced. The nutrition professional can be front and center in this remarkable revolution. Policymakers need to give serious consideration to what policies are necessary at all levels so that we as nutrition professionals can deliver on the promise before us.

Useful Resources

Cordain L, Brand-Miller J, Eaton SB, Mann N, Holt SHA, Speth JD. Plant-animal subsistence ratios and macronutrient energy estimations in worldwide hunter-gatherers. *Am J Clin Nutr.* 2000; 71:682–692.

Eaton SB, Konner M. Paleolithic nutrition. A consideration of its nature and current implications. *N Engl J Med.* 1985; 312:283–289.

Johnson DB, Eaton DL, Wahl PW, Gleason C. Public health nutrition practice in the United States. *J Am Diet Assoc.* 2001; 101:529–534.

Khoury MJ, Burke W, Thomson EJ, eds. *Genetics and Public Health in the 21st Century: Using Genetic Information to Improve Health and Prevent Disease.* New York, NY: Oxford University Press; 2000.

Nordlee JA, Taylor SL, Townsend JA, Thomas LA, Bush RK. Identification of a Brazil-nut allergen in transgenic soybeans. *N Engl J Med.* 1996; 334:688–692.

Taylor SL, Hefle SL. Will genetically modified foods be allergenic? *J Allergy Clin Immunol.* 2001; 107:765–771.

Watkins SM, Hammock BD, Newman JW, German JB. Individual metabolism should guide agriculture toward foods for improved health and nutrition. *Am J Clin Nutr.* 2001; 74:283–286.

Wood AJJ. Racial differences in the response to drugs—pointers to genetic differences. *N Engl J Med.* 2001; 344:1393–1395.

Useful Web Sites

Food and Drug Administration Proposed Rule and Draft Guidance on Labeling Bioengineered Foods

Electronic reading room page. Food and Drug Administration Web site. Available at: http://www.fda.gov/foi/electrr.htm. Accessed August 6, 2002.

Premarket notice concerning bioengineered foods: proposed rule. Food and Drug Administration Web site. Available at: http://www.fda.gov/OHRMS/ DOCKETS/98fr/011801a.htm. Accessed August 6, 2002.

Voluntary labeling indicating whether foods have or have not been developed using bioengineering: draft guidance. Center for Food Safety and Applied Nutrition page. Food and Drug Administration Web site. Available at: http:// vm.cfsan.fda.gov/~dms/biolabgu.html. Accessed August 6, 2002.

General Policy Issues

Agricultural biotechnology: frequently asked questions. Animal and Plant Inspection Service page. Department of Agriculture Web site. Available at: http://www.aphis.usda.gov/ppq/biotech/#FAQ. Accessed August 6, 2002.

Beskow LM, Khoury MJ, Baker TG, Thrasher JF. The integration of genomics into public health research, policy, and practice in the United States: system management. Centers for Disease Control Web site. Available at: http://www.cdc.gov/ genomics/info/reports/research/wheel.htm. Accessed August 6, 2002.

Biotechnology Industry Organization Web site. Available at: http://www.bio.org. Accessed August 6, 2002.

Council for Biotechnology Information Web page. Available at: http:// www.whybiotech.com. Accessed August 6, 2002.

Khoury MJ, Thrasher JF, Burke W, Gettig EA, Fridinger F, Jackson R. Challenges in communicating genetics: a public health approach. Centers for Disease Control Web site. Available at: http://www.cdc.gov/genomics/info/reports/ program/communicate.htm. Accessed August 6, 2002.

National Academy of Sciences. Genetically modified pest-protected plants: science and regulation. April 2000. Available at: http://books.nap.edu/books/ 0309069300/html/l.html. Accessed August 6, 2002.

9

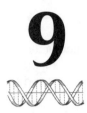

Opportunities for Nutrition Professionals

Genetics may not, at first glance, seem like a direction that would yield obvious expanding opportunities for nutrition professionals, but as we have seen, genetics is the foundation on which medicine is built. Genetics is fundamentally changing health care as we know it, including nutrition therapy, and it will have an equivalent impact on the role of nutrition in health promotion as well as disease prevention and management. As genetics becomes increasingly recognized as a foundational science and more applications become available, there will be a growing need for nutrition professionals with genetics competency. The nutrition professional with a firm command of the field will be in a position to choose among several options for applying that expertise.

OPPORTUNITIES FOR GENETICS-SAVVY NUTRITION PROFESSIONALS

Despite the growing demand, opportunities are not likely to come begging the nutrition professional to take advantage of them. Nutrition professionals are perceived as having knowledge within a fairly limited scope, and genetics expertise is not within that expected scope. It will be up to you to change this perception, which will require a clear vision of where you're going and considerable persistence. Whichever opportunity you choose to pursue, you will need to demonstrate to the client, the health care team, the laboratory, or the manufacturer with whom you are partnering that your nutrition background adds value.

Clinical Practice Opportunities

Beginning with the expansion of conventional opportunities available to nutrition professionals, an obvious application of genetics to nutrition is in clinical practice. The genetics-savvy nutrition professional will analyze the client's family history with an eye toward noticing disorders that occur in the extended family and, knowing how each of these disorders is inherited, will be alert to the patient's risk factors. A major contribution the nutrition professional can make to the health care team is to see the red flags that other practitioners typically miss. It's often the nutrition professional who raises the possibility of gluten-sensitive enteropathy or hemochromatosis, disorders that have a high prevalence within the U.S. population and yet can take five to seven years after onset of symptoms to reach an accurate diagnosis. Understanding that carrier individuals likely have some degree of impairment as a result of having one normal and one faulty gene (the idea of a graded or gene dosage effect), the nutrition professional will predict from the family history that an individual is likely to have subclinical impairment or is at risk for developing such an impairment and will be able to alert the physician to suggest appropriate monitoring or diagnostics.

Writing in the *Journal of the American Medical Association* in 1997, Francis Collins, M.D., Ph.D., Director of the National Human Genome Research Institute (the NIH arm of the Human Genome Project), made the argument that, because of the inadequate number of clinical genetics professionals, the responsibility for using and interpreting genetic diagnostic tests will fall increasingly to primary care physicians. Physicians have at best only a working knowledge of genetics and genetic counseling and, in his opinion, will increasingly need to rely on other members of the health care team to provide genetics expertise. Although Collins had in mind physician assistants, nurses, psychologists, and social workers, the genetics-savvy nutrition professional should be able to fill this role better than any of these other health care professionals. Forming synergistic partnerships between a nutrition professional and, for example, a pharmacist knowledgeable in genetics can provide the physician with a comprehensive approach to the various medical and environmental options available to a client.

Teaching Opportunities

There is a growing need to educate nutrition and other health care professionals as well as the public about genetics and the link with food and nutrition. This education may occur within the formal structure of the academic curriculum or within continuing education programs. For the public, educational opportunities may take a variety of forms, from lectures to print articles to Web postings. Different approaches will be necessary for children and adults.

Undergraduate and graduate nutrition education   Educating the next generation of nutrition professionals about genetics and its connections to food and nutrition is a specialty that will expand at the undergraduate and graduate education levels. The academic preparation of nutrition professionals benefits tremendously from teachers who not only have an excellent grounding in the underlying science of nutrition, but who also have considerable practical experience and, ideally, continue to build that experience by maintaining hands-on laboratory or consulting experience in addition to their teaching responsibilities. Genetics-savvy nutrition professionals will be needed to teach students how genetics is applied to nutrition therapy, medical therapy, and food-related specialties. Those who are actually practicing in the interface between traditional nutrition and genetics will be able to provide students with a vision for emerging opportunities along with practical tips on how to maximize those opportunities.

Continuing professional education   Practicing nutrition professionals as well as health care professionals in general need to be taught the basics of genetics and its relationship to nutrition. Most health care professionals receive minimal education in nutrition. The situation is similar with genetics, which means any education concerning the connection between the two fields is even less likely. A potential stumbling block here is that health care professionals typically want to be taught by someone within their profession and, ideally, by someone within their own area of specialization. The genetics-savvy nutrition professional can overcome this hurdle by being able to communicate valuable information that other health care professionals cannot readily obtain elsewhere. If breaking this barrier is too far beyond your comfort zone, consider partnering with various health care professionals who have access to the audiences that you want to reach.

Public health education   Another opportunity lies with educating the public about genetics in general and how lifestyle choices, most notably nutrition, can influence the expression of the messages encoded in our genes. Many citizens are not science literate; genetics scares them. It is a great service to be able to translate the complexities of genetics into down-to-earth applications that affect everyday life. As genetics is increasingly incorporated into health care, the public health educator will become involved in informing the public about how genetics will affect health care. Educational needs span the range from basic association of genes with disease to new diagnostic tests to the rights of the individual with respect to genetic information.

Diseases–at least the chronic diseases that are the major public health challenges–will likely be found to result primarily from interactions of genes with the environment. Ways to identify susceptible populations will be developed. Susceptibilities will increasingly be linked to modifiable risk factors. Interventions will focus on altering environmental factors, notably nutrition, physical activity, and other lifestyle choices. Public health educators can play a major role in increasing public awareness about the gene-environment connection, the more common triggers of genetic events that lead to disease, and the major health-promoting interventions that can help prevent disease.

As genetics increasingly begins to direct nutrition policy, the public health educator will be involved in implementing nutrition policy that is increasingly personalized and complex. This task will likely challenge even the best communicators. Sound, generalized messages will be necessary, as well as guidelines for tailoring these general recommendations to the individual. Many such messages are already emerging: the folate message for preconception and prenatal care, food safety issues relating to genetically engineered foods, the recent change in dietary guidelines for lowering blood fats that recognizes differing responses to low-fat diets, and the matching of foods by glycemic index to individuals with insulin dysregulation.

Education is needed for adult populations, but also for children, beginning at an early age. Children need to be taught where disease comes from. Many people think a disease is simply caught or that it mysteriously arises from genes deep within the body. Getting the message out that lifestyle choices influence whether or not a disease develops and that people have options they can exercise to influence the outcome of their personal health is a major contribution the public health educator can make.

Research Opportunities

Genetic technologies are increasingly being incorporated into virtually every research laboratory related to either health or agriculture as well as disciplines in between, such as toxicology. There is a potential place for the nutrition professional at every level of expertise, from the holder of a bachelor's degree to the postdoctoral researcher to the principal investigator. If you enjoy the detective work of research, and particularly if you are skilled in the laboratory, consider being part of a scientific research team. Opportunities exist in universities and medical centers as well as in laboratories run by the government or private businesses. Depending on the laboratory, the focus may be basic or applied research. Scientific directors are always looking for competent people with a strong science background who understand the scientific method, can think independently, and have a strong work ethic. There is considerable satisfaction in contributing to solutions that result in improved health care or product development.

Toxicology   One area continually moving in the direction of a nutrition focus is *toxicology*, a field encompassing how environmental signals interact with the genetic material, the impact of this interaction on health, and the ability to change the outcome using nutritional guidelines. The National Institute of Environmental Health Sciences maintains an active and expanding research program focusing on the relationship between environmental influences and gene expression with respect to health and disease. The Environmental Protection Agency also conducts research in toxicology. In addition to having a full complement of staff from a variety of backgrounds, both agencies contract with private companies to conduct research for them. The opportunity exists to work for such companies or even to start a new company and compete for federal contracts.

Biotechnology   In addition to opportunities in the research and development laboratories of biotechnology companies, genetics-savvy nutrition professionals are needed to convert the complex science behind these companies' products into consumer-friendly messages. Recently a biotech company recruiting subjects for a clinical trial of one of its therapeutics wanted a nutrition professional with research experience and an understanding of genetics to participate in the company's presentations to groups of prospective participants. Biotechnology products range from drugs for therapeutic use to nonfood agricultural applications to foods that have been engineered for greater yield or enhanced nutrition. Nutrition professionals can find a niche anywhere, from the basic research required to develop and test these products to the preparation of educational activities and materials needed to increase public understanding of biotechnology and its risks and benefits.

Clinical trial coordinator Organizing and managing clinical trials for testing gene-based therapeutics is yet another research-oriented opportunity for nutrition professionals. A background in clinical practice, research, and genetics is essential. Historically, clinical trial coordinators have been registered nurses who have obtained additional certification as clinical research coordinators, but a nutrition professional with extensive clinical experience would also be a viable candidate. As trials increasingly focus on gene-based therapeutics, the individual with genetics knowledge is likely to have the definitive edge.

Sales Opportunities

Successful salespeople are often excellent educators. Particularly where therapeutic or food products have a strong genetic research and development base, customers will need to rely on the salesperson to be knowledgeable and able to educate them. Nutrition professionals who can bridge the clinical and research aspects of the products presented and apply their formidable people skills to working with customers, who range from physicians to buyers for retail establishments, can expect to succeed in the sales arena.

Genetic Counseling Opportunities

There is a growing demand for genetic counseling, and the number of genetic counselors presently available cannot adequately meet even the current, let alone the projected, demand. For those who enjoy counseling, marrying genetic counseling and nutrition therapy makes sense. Traditionally, the genetic counselor has been primarily involved with prenatal diagnosis and pediatrics. Now that our understanding of the genetic basis of disease has expanded considerably, genetic counselors are increasingly in demand in preventive health care.

The genetic counselor plays a valuable role as both teacher and counselor. Working with a board-certified geneticist, he or she helps to identify families at risk and educates them about their particular disorder, the genetic testing involved, the interpretations of the test results, and the medical options available. The genetic counselor is an important link between the physician and the family. Many families do not understand how a disease is inherited and how its presence will affect their lives; they therefore benefit immeasurably from the skills of a genetic counselor.

Consider combining your nutrition background with training in genetic counseling for a unique combination of skills. In addition to identifying family members at risk for a particular disorder, you would be able to counsel them on nutritional approaches that can help prevent the development of the disorder. For those members who have already developed the disorder, you'll move beyond the limitations of genetic counseling and offer nutritional interventions that can minimize the negative impact of the disorder on their quality of life.

Genetic counselors are master's-level professionals who have completed a two-year training program that includes a practicum and have passed a national certification exam. Certification in genetic counseling is available through the American Board of Genetic Counseling (see "Useful Web Sites" section below for Web address). There are several training programs in the United States and Canada. Typical coursework includes a solid foundation in human genetics (clinical genetics, population genetics, cytogenetics, biochemical, and molecular genetics) coupled with psychosocial theory, ethics, and counseling techniques. The clinical practicum is an integral part of the degree requirements and takes place in medical genetics centers.

PREPARING FOR THE GENETIC REVOLUTION

To take advantage of these opportunities, we must become genetics-savvy nutrition professionals. All nutrition professionals today, regardless of focus, need to develop a strong and broad-based science foundation in order to maximize the many opportunities emerging. A solid science base is even more important when adding genetics competency to your skills, because genetics cuts across so many disciplines within health care. Although it's more challenging to learn a new discipline once you have left the academic environment and are working full-time, nutrition professionals can develop competency in genetics at all stages of their careers.

Academic Preparation

Take the hard road whenever possible, which means science courses intended for majors rather than the science-for-allied-health-professionals track. You want to ground yourself thoroughly in the basic sciences and position yourself as flexibly as possible in a rapidly changing world in which new scientific discoveries and applications are commonplace. We cannot begin to imagine where science will take us in five, ten, or twenty years. Do not shortchange your career options—build the strongest foundation you can.

A solid foundation includes chemistry (including inorganic, organic, and biochemistry), physics, biology (basic plant biology, cell biology, microbiology, anatomy and physiology, and genetics), and food science and nutrition (food science, metabolism, and diet therapy). For your genetics selections, take at least a basic genetics lecture and an experimental lab to learn the rudiments of research. Try to get some experience in a genetics research laboratory, either as part of a work-study program or as a directed individual study with a genetics-oriented professor. Genetic risk is discussed in terms of probability, and genetic knowledge accumulates through experimentation and the use of research studies. Thus a basic understanding of statistics and research design is also necessary.

Following your undergraduate preparation, select a master's program in genetics or genetic counseling. Genetics programs will emphasize research and, depending on which university and research laboratory you choose, can direct you toward basic research, food applications, clinical trials, private industry, or teaching. Genetic counseling programs focus on clinical genetics and on working with individuals and families at risk for disease.

Even if you have been out of school awhile, you don't have to be left behind. Learning is a lifelong process, and it's never too late to learn something new. The current situation with genetics is analogous to the computer revolution. Those of us who started to slowly educate ourselves twenty years ago when computers entered the mass market are comfortable with today's computer-based society—so it will be with the genetics revolution. If you are fortunate enough to live near a university, taking a basic course in genetics is a great way to start. Self-study is another viable option. Distance learning will soon bring genetics to you. The information is available—master it and make it work for you to open new opportunities.

Incorporating Genetics into Your Career

Begin to arm yourself with the skills you will need to be comfortable with genetics. Learn the language. Begin to think about how genetics can fit into your career path and unique interests. Explore the additional education and training necessary for the particular aspect of the genetics-nutrition combination that interests you.

It's not necessary to wait until you have become a genetics expert to begin to incorporate genetics and genetic-directed thinking into your current position. If you are in clinical practice, incorporate a detailed family history into your assessments. Learn to look for red flags within that history and alert the physician so that effective therapies can be developed for the patient and family members. Select a disease among the ones that you encounter most frequently and learn how that disease is inherited (which will give you clues as to who in the patient's family is also at risk). Learn about the genes responsible for that disease, and find out whether there are environmental and lifestyle factors involved that you might be able to help the patient manipulate to ameliorate the disorder or prevent its expression. What research is currently being conducted relating to this gene-disease association? Just reading the studies published will often help you focus on where you need to start in learning the language and understanding the techniques used.

If you work in public health, begin to think about how genetics will affect your field. How will genetics allow you to become more effective at preventing disease? What health promotion messages will be effective? Most likely your audience, the public, knows no more about genetics than you do. As you prepare yourself for the genetic revolution, think about how many questions the public will have and what helped you understand the important concepts. Can you convert your experience into teaching tools for educating the public? If you work with the Women, Infants, and Children (WIC) program, it's particularly important to identify disease susceptibility early and begin nutritional interventions. Again, collecting family data can help identify other family members who would benefit from education and intervention.

At the very least, each of us needs to be able to do the following:

- Engage in intelligent conversation with a physician or other health care professional who stops us in the hallway and wants to discuss an article he or she has read in a professional journal relating to genetics and nutrition
- Read a genetics study and understand what was done and its implications
- Answer questions from clients reading today's health-related headlines and news stories
- Be knowledgeable enough to decide when we have enough information to begin incorporating genetics into our work

At most, those interested in advanced practice opportunities that combine genetics and nutrition should develop a solid foundation in genetics and in how nutrition and genetics integrate into effective therapeutic options, as well as consider obtaining advanced training in genetics and nutrition. This career path may include pursuing advanced degrees in genetics or genetic counseling, research opportunities linking genetics and nutrition, or certification in a genetics-nutrition specialty yet to be developed.

The potential rewards for expanding our careers to include genetics are considerable. Having a combination of skills in a growing market positions the nutrition professional for a considerably higher income than we typically command. Job satisfaction is high because adding the genetic perspective to nutrition practice can produce highly effective outcomes, which translates into healthy, satisfied patients as well as increased respect for the nutrition professional's valuable expertise. This positions us as essential members of the health care team.

Useful Resources

American Board of Genetic Counseling (ABGC), 9650 Rockville Pike, Bethesda, Md 20894–3998, Ph: 301/571-1825; Fax: 301/571-1895 Web site available at: http://www.abgc.net

Bowers DF, Allred J. Advances in molecular biology: implications for the future of clinical nutrition practice. *J Am Diet Assoc.* 1995; 95:53–59.

Collins FS. Preparing health care professionals for the genetic revolution. *JAMA.* 1997; 278:1285–1286.

Mahabir S, Berwick M. What dietetics can learn from molecular biology. *J Am Diet Assoc.* 1995; 95:748.

Patterson RE, Eaton DL, Potter JD. The genetic revolution: change and challenge for the dietetics profession. *J Am Diet Assoc.* 1999; 99:1412–1420.

Useful Web Sites

Association of Professors of Human and Medical Genetics/American Society of Human Genetics. Medical School Core Curriculum in Genetics. *Am J Hum Genet.* 1995; 56:535–537. Available at: http://www.faseb.org/genetics/ashg/policy/rep-01.htm. Accessed August 6, 2002.

Clinical genetic education resources (courses and lectures). University of Kansas Medical Center Web site. Available at: http://www.kumc.edu/gec/prof/genecour.html. Accessed August 6, 2002.

Genetics Education and Counseling Program. University of Pittsburgh Web site. Available at: http://www.pitt.edu/~edugene. Accessed August 6, 2002.

Genomics competencies for the public health workforce. CDC Web site. Available at: http://www.cdc.gov/genomics/training/competencies/comps.htm. Accessed August 6, 2002.

Human Genome Project information: genetic counseling Department of Energy Web site. Available at: http://www.ornl.gov/hgmis/medicine/genecounseling.html. Accessed August 6, 2002.

Johnson VP, Christianson C. Clinical genetics: a self study for health care providers lesson 2: taking a family history. Virtual Hospital Web site. Available at: http://www.vh.org/Providers/Textbooks/ClinicalGenetics/Lesson2/FamHistory.html. Accessed August 6, 2002, December 27, 2001.

Medical genetics: recommended core educational guidelines for family practice residents. *Am Fam Physician* [serial online]. 1999; 60(1):305–308. Available at: http://www.aafp.org. Accessed August 6, 2002.

National Coalition for Health Professional Education in Genetics. Core competencies in genetics essential for all health-care professionals. February 14, 2000. Available at: http://www.nchpeg.org/core/core.asp. Accessed August 6, 2002.

National Institute of Environmental Health Sciences Web site. Available at: http://www.niehs.nih.gov. Accessed August 6, 2002.

ResourceLink: genetic counseling resources. National Society of Genetic Counselors Web site. Available at: http://www.nsgc.org/resourcelink.asp. Accessed August 6, 2002.

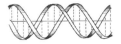

Glossary

Adenine (A)   A nitrogenous base, one of the four that make up a nucleic acid sequence (DNA or RNA); its complementary base-pairing partner in DNA is thymine (T) and in RNA is uracil (U).

Allele   The different forms (DNA sequences) that a gene may have; one allele is inherited from each parent.

Amino acid   Any of a class of twenty different nitrogen-containing molecules that join together to form a protein (or a polypeptide in the case of a protein with multiple polypeptide subunits); each amino acid in the protein is specified by a codon in the DNA sequence that codes for that protein.

Amniocentesis   A prenatal diagnostic test in which fetal cells shed into the amniotic fluid are removed; the chromosomes are examined for defects in size and number and the DNA can be analyzed for particular diseases. Amniocentesis is performed in the second trimester of pregnancy, approximately sixteen weeks after the last menstrual period.

Amplification   See *DNA amplification.*

Animal model   An animal used as a model organism for genetic and other research involving human biochemistry and physiology.

Annotation   A term often used to describe the next phase of the Human Genome Project, whereby details will be associated with the raw DNA sequence information, such as the gene coded for, the amino acid sequence coded for, the function of the protein produced, and so on.

Antibody   A protein produced by plasma cells of the animal immune system in response to the presence of an antigen; antibodies neutralize invading microorganisms or foreign proteins by binding to antigens on their surfaces.

Anticodon   A three-nucleotide sequence on each transfer RNA (tRNA) molecule that attaches to messenger RNA (mRNA) through complementary base pairing during translation of the mRNA into the amino acid sequence of the protein; the anticodon pairing ensures the correct amino acid is inserted at the proper position in protein synthesis.

Antigen   A substance considered to be foreign to an animal's immune system that induces an immune response in which antibodies functioning against it are produced.

Antisense technology   A strategy for preventing the synthesis of a protein; a nucleic acid fragment is constructed whose sequence is complementary to that of a messenger RNA sequence. Binding of the antisense sequence prevents the mRNA from being translated into protein.

Apoptosis   Programmed cell death; organisms dispose of damaged cells through the process of apoptosis.

Autosomal   A term describing how a trait is inherited; if the gene that determines the trait resides on an autosome, the pattern of inheritance will follow the rules of distribution for autosomes.

Autosomal dominant   A mode of inheritance in which a trait carried on one of the twenty-two autosome pairs is expressed even if only one copy of the gene determining that trait is defective (mutated).

Autosomal recessive   A mode of inheritance in which a trait carried on one of the twenty-two autosome pairs is not expressed unless both copies of the gene determining the trait are defective (mutated).

Autosomes   Those chromosomes that do not determine sex; in human beings the autosomes are the chromosome pairs numbered 1 through 22.

BAC (bacterial artificial chromosome)   A type of bacterial cloning vector; this recombinant plasmid originally from the bacterium *Escherichia coli* can accept an insert of foreign DNA of approximately 150 base pairs.

Bacillus thuringiensis **(Bt)**   A bacterium that normally lives in the soil; Bt has been used for many years by farmers and home gardeners to ward off pests. When ingested by a pest, the Bt protein toxin disrupts the pest's digestive system.

Base   One of the four building blocks of the DNA and RNA molecules of all life forms; all bases contain nitrogen. The four bases of DNA are adenine (A), cytosine (C), guanine (G), and thymine (T). The four bases of RNA are adenine (A), cytosine (C), guanine (G), and uracil (U). There are two classes of bases: purines (adenine, guanine) and pyrimidines (cytosine, thymine, and uracil).

Base pair   Two bases on opposite strands in double-stranded DNA that are held together weakly by hydrogen bonds in a process called complementary base pairing. Adenine (A) binds with thymine (T) and cytosine (C) binds with guanine (G). The base pairing holds the two strands of DNA together in its characteristic double helix.

Base pair substitution   A type of mutation in which one of the DNA bases is replaced with another DNA base.

Base sequence   The order in which bases occur on a segment of DNA or any of the RNA molecules.

Base sequence analysis   See *DNA sequencing.*

Bioinformatics   The relatively new science of using computers to manage and analyze the vast amount of information being generated by the Human Genome Project.

Biotechnology   The use of living organisms to make products or perform therapeutic services; the primary technologies for modern-day biotechnology have been recombinant DNA technology and monoclonal antibody technology.

bp   Abbreviation for *Base pair.*

BRCA1/BRCA2   Mutations associated with breast cancer.

Buccal swab   A noninvasive procedure of obtaining a DNA sample whereby cells are gently scraped from the inside of the cheek (buccal cavity).

Cancer   Uncontrolled cell growth; normal cell growth gone awry.

Carrier   A heterozygote–an individual who has one copy of a normal gene and one copy of a mutant gene; from a health perspective, the mutation may increase or decrease the risk of developing a particular condition. Whether or not the health of the carrier is affected by this mutant gene depends on the nature of the mutation and its impact on function, but carriers can pass the mutant gene along to their children.

cDNA   Abbreviation for *Complementary DNA.*

Celera Genomics   Private company headed by J. Craig Venter, Ph.D., that has played a major role in the Human Genome Project in determining the sequencing of the human genome.

Cell   The basic subunit of a living organism; most cells contain a nucleus, inside which is the genetic material.

Cell fusion   Formation of a cell by joining the nuclei of two or more different cell types; cell fusion is often used when generating transgenic plants and animals or when introducing a DNA sequence from one cell into another.

Centimorgan (cM)   Unit of measurement of recombination frequency; centimorgans are used to describe the distance between markers on a genetic linkage map.

Centromere   A specialized region of a chromosome to which the spindle fibers attach during cell division and that helps to ensure the chromosomes are distributed correctly to the daughter cells.

Chorionic villus sampling (CVS)   A prenatal test during the first trimester of pregnancy that involves examining cells surrounding the fetus to look for defects in the chromosomes of these cells and to analyze the DNA for particular disorders.

Chromosome   Made of DNA and protein; a way to package all the DNA into discrete amounts rather than having one long molecule; human beings have 46 chromosomes, found in the nucleus of a cell. A particular gene has a specific location on one of the chromosomes. Except for the X and Y chromosomes in the male, they occur in pairs.

Chromosome painting   A diagnostic technique whereby probes with different-colored fluorescent dyes hybridize to the chromosomes of a cell to determine whether the structure of the chromosomes is normal or whether changes have occurred.

Clone   An exact copy of biological material; a clone may be a DNA sequence, a gene, a cell, or an organism. When referring to cells, it is a group of cells derived from a single ancestor.

Cloning   Making an exact copy of something, whether a DNA sequence, a gene, or an organism. See also *DNA cloning, Gene cloning.*

Cloning vector   A DNA molecule that originated with a bacterium, a virus, or the cell of a higher organism, into which can be inserted a segment of DNA that will subsequently be copied each time the host cell duplicates its DNA; vectors are used to introduce foreign DNA into a host cell. Examples include plasmids, human artificial chromosomes, yeast artificial chromosomes, and various viruses.

cM   Abbreviation for *Centimorgan.*

Codominance   A condition in which both alleles are expressed when present in the heterozygous state; an example is the AB blood type, in which both the A antigen and the B antigen are expressed and appear on the surface of blood cells.

Codon   A set of three nucleotide bases in DNA that specifies an amino acid or represents a signal to start or stop transcription.

Comparative genomics   Analyzing DNA sequences of human beings and several model systems; because of the similarity between human beings and many other organisms in terms of genes carried in the genomes and the similar functions of these genes, using knowledge of genes from other organisms has been a powerful strategy for identifying human genes and interpreting their functions.

Complementary base pairing   The weak hydrogen bonding between bases in double-stranded nucleic acids; this pairing can occur with DNA, in which adenine pairs with thymine and guanine with cytosine, or it can occur between DNA and mRNA or between mRNA and tRNA, in which adenine pairs with uracil and guanine with cytosine.

Complementary DNA (cDNA)   Single-stranded DNA synthesized to complement the base sequence of messenger RNA (mRNA) and often used as a probe; cDNA contains exons but no introns.

Complementary sequences   Single-stranded nucleic acid base sequences that can form a double-stranded structure by matching the base pairs of the sequences (hybridizing).

Congenital   Existing at the time of birth.

Conserved DNA sequences   Sequences of DNA that have remained relatively unchanged throughout evolution; they are thought to be associated with important functions that are similar in different species, since unrelated species share many of the same conserved sequences.

Conserved protein sequences   Amino acid sequences found in protein that have remained essentially unchanged throughout evolution.

Contigs   Groups of clones that represent overlapping regions of a genome.

Crossing over   Part of the gene shuffling that occurs when new organisms are created; the maternal and paternal chromosomes pair along their length during meiosis, when sperm and egg cells are formed. During this time, the chromosomes can exchange sections with their partners. Crossing over thereby increases the variability of genetic information because the maternal member of the pair now contains some of the paternal genetic information and vice versa. This exchange of genetic information is the basis for variability even among siblings from the same parents.

Cytogenetic testing   Examination of the chromosomes of an individual to check that the correct number is present and that structure of each is normal.

Cytokines   Protein growth factors, such as interleukins, interferons, and tumor necrosis factors involved in the inflammatory response, causing cells to proliferate.

Cytosine (C)   A nitrogenous base, one of the four that make up a nucleic acid sequence (DNA or RNA); its complementary base pairing partner is guanine (G).

Deletion   A type of mutation in which genetic information has been lost; the loss may involve a single base or an entire chromosome.

Deoxyribonucleic acid (DNA)   The molecule that contains the genetic information (the blueprint for development and function) of living organisms; in higher organisms, DNA is found in the nucleus of cells.

Diploid   Having a full set of genetic information, one set of chromosomes from each parent; most animal cells except sperm and egg cells contain a diploid set of chromosomes. In human beings the diploid number of chromosomes is 46.

DNA   Abbreviation for *Deoxyribonucleic acid.*

DNA amplification   The process of making multiple copies of a DNA sequence; amplification may occur in vivo using a cloning vector or in vitro through a polymerase chain reaction (PCR).

DNA array   See *DNA microarray.*

DNA-based testing   The use of DNA probes to detect the presence of a mutation.

DNA cloning   A technique of genetic engineering whereby a segment of DNA is taken from one organism and moved into another organism, often for the purposes of making more of a product specified by a particular gene; for example, the gene for human insulin was cloned into a bacterium, which multiplies rapidly and produces insulin in the process.

DNA marker   See *Marker.*

DNA microarray   A detection system that tells which genes are switched on in a given cell; only a small fraction of the total genetic material is being actively expressed at any given time, and microarray technology detects that material.

DNA polymerase   Enzyme that copies DNA and repairs it; it uses one strand of DNA to synthesize the complementary copy.

DNA probe   A sequence of single-stranded DNA used to detect a complementary sequence of single-stranded DNA; probes are labeled with a detectable substance, usually radioactivity or a fluorescent dye, so that the target DNA sequence to which the probe has bound can be detected.

DNA replication   The process by which DNA is duplicated; replication requires the enzyme DNA polymerase, which uses one strand of DNA as a template to synthesize the new strand through complementary base pairing.

DNA sequencing   A method for determining the base sequence of DNA; it is ultimately expected to become an automatic process in wide use.

DNA typing   Similar to blood typing, only far more specific; using DNA to generate the unique genetic fingerprint for an individual for the purpose of identifying him or her unequivocally, since no one else except an identical twin can have the exact same DNA.

Dominant   A gene whose effect is expressed; this is usually the normal form of a gene, but with certain defective genes, the defect is expressed and dominates the normal form (compare *Recessive*).

Double helix   The shape that two strands of DNA assume when they are bonded together through complementary base pairing; it resembles a spiral staircase.

Double-stranded DNA   The normal configuration for DNA; two strands of the genetic material are held together by complementary base pairing.

Electrophoresis   A method of separating a mixture of large molecules, such as DNA fragments or proteins; an electric current is passed through a gel matrix containing the mixture, and the components are physically separated based on their size or electrical charge. Agarose and acrylamide are the gels commonly used.

Embryonic stem cells   Early embryonic cells that have not yet differentiated; they can be genetically manipulated and then implanted into embryos to produce transgenic animals with specific genetic traits.

Endonuclease   An enzyme that can cut nucleotides at specific locations within the nucleic acid sequence (compare *Exonuclease*). See also *Restriction enzymes.*

Environment   The nongenetic factors that influence gene expression and ultimately an individual's health and well-being.

Enzyme   Protein molecule that facilitates the conversion of one substance into another; it is critical for all aspects of cell growth and metabolism.

EST   Abbreviation for *Expressed sequence tag.*

Eukaryote   An organism that has a nucleus, a membrane-bound, structurally distinct, subcellular compartment that houses the genetic material; cells from these organisms are often described as eukaryotic cells. All organisms except bacteria and blue-green algae are eukaryotes. Also spelled *eucaryote* (compare *Prokaryote*).

Evolution   The process by which all life-forms change incrementally over time due to the need to adapt to their changing environment; the basis for evolution is the introduction of DNA variation and the passage of this variation from one generation to the next.

Exon   The protein-coding DNA sequences within a gene; in most genes exons are separated by introns, segments of DNA that do not code for proteins. The introns are removed in the process of producing mature messenger RNA so that only the exons remain to direct the synthesis of the protein coded for by that gene.

Exonuclease   An enzyme that cleaves nucleotides sequentially from the free ends of the nucleotide segment, rather than cleaving within the segment (compare *Endonuclease*).

Expression   The ability to retrieve the encoded genetic information in the DNA and convert it first into messenger RNA and then into the proteins that do the work of the cells; it also refers to whether a trait that results from an error in DNA information is manifested.

Expressed gene   A segment of DNA transcribed into messenger RNA.

Expressed sequence tag (EST)   A sequence tagged site (STS) derived from cDNA; it is used as a landmark when developing the physical map of the human genome. ESTs represent portions of expressed genes.

Extrachromosomal DNA   DNA that is separate from the main chromosome; in bacteria this DNA is usually a plasmid, a small, self-replicating, circular piece of DNA that has been very useful as a cloning vector.

Fermentation   The process of growing microorganisms for the production of various gene products, such as therapeutic proteins; this process is used in biotechnology to scale up from the laboratory to the large quantities of material needed for commercial production.

FISH   Abbreviation for *Fluorescent in situ hybridization.*

Flow cytometry   The process of using a laser beam to analyze the light-absorbing or fluorescein-emitting properties of biological material such as cells or subcellular components such as chromosomes to generate a profile of this material; it can be used to analyze the chromosomes in cells and to sort chromosomes so that multiple copies of a single chromosome can be collected and used for studies investigating its composition.

Flow karyotyping   The process of using flow cytometry to separate chromosomes based on their DNA content; this process can be automated to construct a karyotype for an individual.

Fluorescent in situ hybridization   A process in which DNA probes are tagged with a fluorescein dye that allows them to be detected when they bind to a region of a chromosome; this process is used to physically map a gene to a chromosome and to analyze whether a cell has the correct number of chromosomes in the normal structural arrangement.

Gamete   Male or female reproductive cell (sperm or egg); each contains a haploid set of chromosomes, which includes twenty-three chromosomes in human beings (one copy from each of the twenty-three pairs).

Gene   A unit of hereditary information; a section within DNA that has a function, such as encoding the information for making a protein.

Gene cloning   The process of making an exact copy of a gene's DNA sequence.

Gene expression   The process of converting the information encoded in the DNA into RNA (mRNA, tRNA, rRNA); most genes are transcribed into mRNA and ultimately into a protein product.

Gene library   A set of clones that collectively represent the entire genome of an organism; restriction enzymes are used to cut the total DNA into overlapping fragments, which are then physically separated and cloned into a vector to amplify the number of copies of the fragment. The clones can be examined with a DNA probe to locate which clone contains the gene of interest. Also called a genomic library.

Gene mapping   Determining the relative positions of genes on DNA molecules (which may come from a chromosome or a vector). This process physically locates a gene at a particular site on a chromosome.

Gene pool   The sum total of all the genes in a particular population.

Gene product   The material that results from the expression of a gene; the end product may be an RNA molecule (mRNA, tRNA, rRNA) or, in the case of mRNA, a protein.

Gene therapy   The process of transferring a normal gene into an organism in order to replace or repair a malfunctioning gene, essentially changing the genetic makeup of an organism to improve its function.

Genetic code   A term referring to the fact that DNA contains the information that dictates which amino acid is inserted into the protein to be synthesized and at which position; the code is read in sets (called codons) of three nucleotides. Each codon corresponds to an amino acid or a start or stop signal. The genetic code is universal, meaning that the lowest form of life uses the same key as the highest form of life, and somewhat redundant, meaning that some amino acids have more than one codon that translates into that particular amino acid.

Genetic counseling Interpretation of DNA testing by individuals specially trained in understanding what the test results mean in terms of disease risk and in helping patients and their families handle the positive and negative impacts of the results.

Genetic determinism The belief that genes control destiny, that whatever information is in a person's genes seals the person's fate.

Genetic disease A disease caused by one or more mutations in the genetic material; mutations may be inherited or arise spontaneously. Contrary to popular usage, genetic disease is not a special category of disease because virtually all diseases have one or more genetic mutations underlying their development, with the exception of infectious disease, which itself is influenced by the genetic makeup of the individual.

Genetic engineering The process of altering the composition and thereby the functioning of the original genetic sequence in a given organism by introducing new genetic material; in this process, genes are removed from, modified in, or added to a living organism. Also called gene splicing. See also *Recombinant DNA technology.*

Genetic linkage map A map giving the relative physical positions of genes or other markers on a chromosome; this map is used to convey the chromosomal location of genes, the order of genes along a chromosome, and the distance between genes on the same chromosome. Such distance is measured in centimorgans (cM).

Genetic marker See *Marker.*

Genetic profile The genetic fingerprint unique to an individual, shared by no one except an identical sibling; this collection of information about an individual's genes and the functional capabilities coded for by those genes can be used to predict such characteristics as responsiveness to drugs, disease susceptibility, and so on.

Genetic screening Large-scale testing of a population to identify people at risk for a specific disorder.

Genetic testing Analyzing DNA to determine whether someone carries the gene that leads to a particular disease such as Huntington's or sickle cell disease; some tests are conducted prenatally to determine whether the fetus has a genetic problem, whereas others are performed postnatally to predict risk of developing a particular disease.

Genetics The science of studying the information stored in the genes of an organism: how the information is stored, how it is retrieved, how that information determines the structure and function of the cells that make up the organism, which factors influence the expression of the genes and the activity of their products, and how they accomplish this influence.

Genome The sum total of all the genetic information in an organism; its genome is its instruction book–the blueprint that directs the development and functioning of an organism, including human beings.

Genomic imprinting The process whereby a trait is expressed differently depending on whether it is inherited from the mother or from the father; examples include Prader-Willi and Angelman syndromes as well as myotonic dystrophy.

Genomic library See *Gene library.*

Genomics Called the "new" genetics; whereas genetics unraveled the one gene–one polypeptide understanding of genes, function, and disease, genomics is a more global view of genetics and focuses on more complex issues such as the interaction of multiple genes on function, protein-protein interactions, and gene-environment interactions.

Genotype The genetic makeup of an individual; the genotype is in opposition to the phenotype, the physiological makeup that results from the expression of the individual's genes, the translation of the genotype information into how an individual looks and functions. When referring to a single locus, genotype refers to the allelic constitution at that particular locus (compare *Phenotype*).

Germ cell   Cells involved in reproduction; in human beings, germ cells give rise to either sperm or egg cells.

Germ line therapy   Altering the genetic information in the germ cells such that successive generations will inherit the modified information and have altered (presumably improved) function.

Guanine (G)   Nitrogenous base, one of four that makes up a nucleic acid sequence (DNA or RNA); its complementary base-pairing partner is cytosine (C).

Haploid   Having half of the full set of genetic information of an organism; in human beings, this amounts to twenty-three chromosomes (one from each pair). Reproductive cells (egg and sperm) contain a haploid set of genetic information (compare *Diploid*).

Haploinsufficiency   Condition whereby 50% of the normal level of gene expression, as occurs in a heterozygous individual, is inadequate for carrying out the full function needed by the individual; in other words, the carrier individual's function is impaired by not having two copies of a normal gene. An example of haploinsufficiency is familial hypercholesterolemia, which causes a deficiency in LDL-cholesterol receptor activity. Heterozygotes have half the normal activity, but this level is not sufficient to control serum cholesterol levels, and these individuals typically have cholesterol levels approximately twice those of normal individuals.

Heredity   The transmission of traits though the genes from parents to offspring.

Heterozygote (adj. heterozygous)   Case in which the two copies of a gene are genetically different; that is, two different alleles are present. A heterozygous individual is also called a carrier (compare *Homozygote*).

Homologues/homologous chromosomes   The two members of a chromosome pair.

Homology (adj. homologous)   Similarities in nucleotide base sequence between two DNA segments or in amino acid sequence between two proteins. This term is used when comparing sequences between individuals of the same species or between species.

Homozygote (adj. homozygous)   Condition in which both alleles of a gene—one on one member of the pair of chromosomes and the other on the second member of the pair—are the same (compare *Heterozygote*).

Human artificial chromosome (HAC)   A synthetic chromosome made in the laboratory that has the basic hallmarks of a chromosome (such as a centromere and telomeres) and a sequence of DNA (usually five to ten thousand base pairs).

Human Genome Project   International effort to identify all of the DNA bases in the human genome and to apply this information to improve health.

Hybridization   The generation of offspring from two genetically dissimilar parents, which can refer to animals, plants, or cells; this term also refers to the process of reannealing DNA, whereby the two single strands find their complementary base-pairing partners and zip together like teeth in a zipper, or of single-stranded DNA and messenger RNA undergoing base pairing to generate a double-stranded hybrid.

Hybridoma   The cell produced from fusing two cells of different origins; a hybridoma is an immortal hybrid antibody-producing cell made by fusing white blood cells and multiple myeloma cells. It secretes a single type of monoclonal antibody.

Imprinting, genomic   See *Genomic imprinting.*

Inheritance   The process by which genes and the traits associated with those genes are passed from generation to generation; Mendelian (traditional) inheritance is readily correlated with the chromosome on which the gene is located (whether autosome, X chromosome, or Y chromosome) and whether the expression of the gene is dominant or recessive. Nontraditional inheritance refers to modes of transmission that are non-Mendelian, such as mitochondrial inheritance, genomic imprinting, uniparental disomy, and possibly other modes that have not yet been determined.

Insertion   A type of mutation in which one or more nucleotide bases have been added to the DNA sequence.

In situ hybridization   The process by which a labeled probe of a DNA sequence complementary to a specific gene binds to a particular region on a chromosome, thereby locating the position of that gene on that chromosome.

International Human Genome Sequencing Consortium   A global team of scientists working together to determine the sequence of the human genome.

Intron   Sequences of nucleotide bases within a gene that do not code for meaningful information and interrupt the coding sequences that contain the information for constructing a protein; introns are removed from messenger RNA before it is translated into the final protein product.

In vitro   Outside a living organism; in the laboratory.

In vitro fertilization (IVF)   Process by which sperm and egg cells are united in the laboratory and the fertilized egg is then implanted into the womb.

In vivo   Inside a living organism.

Junk DNA   Those stretches of nucleotide bases between genes that originally did not appear to code for useful information; noncoding DNA makes up approximately 99% of the entire human genome. Findings from the Human Genome Project, however, suggest that these sequences may indeed be of consequence.

Karyotype   A form of analysis in which chromosomes are isolated from cells of an individual or fetus and arranged in picture form from largest to smallest. This analysis provides information about the number of chromosomes, their size, and some information as to whether the genetic information is in the correct order typical for each chromosome.

Kilobase (kb)   A measurement of the length of a DNA fragment equal to one thousand nucleotides (base pairs).

Knockout mice   Experimental mice in which the function of one or more genes has been eliminated so that the researcher can study the effect of the loss of that function.

Library   A set of DNA fragments that has been cloned, one fragment per clone; these fragments are unordered and do not necessarily collectively represent the entire genome of an organism (compare *Gene library*).

Ligase   A category of enzyme that can splice DNA segments together; ligases are important in biotechnology for joining DNA segments from different sources.

Linkage   The physical proximity of two or more markers along the DNA; the closer together the markers are, the greater the probability they will be inherited together. Such markers are said to be linked; linkage analysis will exhibit less than 50% recombination (compare *Linkage Analysis*).

Linkage analysis   Genetic manipulation designed to measure whether two or more markers are located physically close to each other within the genome. The offspring of a mating are analyzed to compare the frequency of occurrence of the parental combination of traits and nonparental (new) combinations of traits; if two genes are linked, the parental combination will occur in 50% or more of the offspring. See also *Recombination.*

Linkage map   See *Genetic linkage map.*

Locus (plural loci)   The actual physical position of a gene or marker on a chromosome; also the DNA sequence at that position.

Mapping   The process of physically locating a gene or marker on a chromosome; the detail of the information varies depending on the genetic analysis (linkage map, physical map).

Marker   An identifiable segment of DNA whose physical location on a particular chromosome is known; its inheritance can be tracked, making it a useful tool for genetic analysis. For example, a gene of interest may have no identifiable characteristic that allows its inheritance to be monitored, but it may lie close to a marker that can be tracked (that is, it may have linkage to the marker)–the marker provides an indirect method of tracking the gene of interest until an assay for its direct detection can be devised.

Maternal inheritance   See *Mitochondrial inheritance*; compare *Mendelian inheritance.*

Meiosis   Specialized cell division of gamete formation in which the diploid set of chromosomes is reduced to a haploid set, one member of each chromosome pair being present in the generated sperm and egg cells.

Mendelian inheritance   The traditional mode of inheritance, whereby the inheritance of traits can be predicted based on whether the gene responsible for the trait is located on an autosome or a sex chromosome and whether its expression is dominant or recessive.

Messenger RNA (mRNA)   The RNA that serves as the template for protein synthesis; genes are expressed in a stepwise process leading ultimately to a protein in most cases. The first step involves converting the information stored in DNA into a messenger RNA molecule that can then be translated into the protein.

Metaphase   Phase of meiosis or mitosis in which the chromosomes are fully condensed and can be made readily visible by staining or other dye treatment.

Microarray technology   A term referring to the ability to test hundreds to thousands of genes at one time; an identical sample of cDNA is dotted onto a glass plate multiple times and labeled probes of sample DNA are then allowed to hybridize to detect whether a DNA complementary to the probe's sequence is present in the sample being tested. Also called gene chip technology.

Microorganism   Any organism that can be seen only through a microscope.

Microsatellite DNA   DNA that consists of small repeat units of three to six base pairs in length; this DNA is particularly useful for identification technology.

Minisatellite DNA   DNA that consists of tandem repeat units ranging in size from twenty to seventy base pairs; variation in the number of repeats is the basis for VNTR polymorphisms. These units are used in DNA typing for identification purposes.

Mitochondrial DNA   Circular DNA that serves as the genetic material of the mitochondria, subcellular organelles involved in cellular respiration.

Mitochondrial inheritance   A nontraditional mode of inheritance whereby genes that reside on the mitochondria are inherited only from the mother. Also called maternal inheritance.

Mitosis   The process of nuclear division that generates daughter cells genetically identical to each other and to the parent.

Molecular testing   See *DNA-based testing.*

Monoclonal antibody   A specialized antibody that is derived from only a single clone of cells and that recognizes only one region of one antigen.

Monogenic   A term that describes a single-gene trait.

Mouse model   A term referring to the use of the genetically defined laboratory mouse as an experimental system in which questions can be asked about genes and their functions and the results lay the foundation for understanding human gene function.

Multifactorial   A term describing traits or diseases that result from the interaction of genes and environmental factors.

Multigenic   A term describing traits or diseases that result from the contribution of more than one gene.

Mutation   A permanent change in the DNA that can be inherited.

Myeloma   A tumor cell, arising from the bone marrow, that is used in monoclonal antibody technology to form hybridomas; the myeloma confers immortality on the hybridoma.

National Human Genome Research Institute   Publicly funded consortium whose mission is the sequencing of the human genome and the genomes of various organisms used as model systems in research laboratories.

Nontraditional genetics   Refers to the inheritance of traits by mechanisms other than Mendelian inheritance, such as mitochondrial inheritance, genomic imprinting, and uniparental disomy.

Nucleic acid   A large polymer of nucleotide subunits; examples are DNA and RNA.

Nucleotide   The building block of nucleic acids, both DNA and RNA; consists of one nitrogenous base, one sugar molecule (deoxyribose for DNA, ribose for RNA), and one phosphate molecule; in DNA the base is adenine, thymine, guanine, or cytosine; in RNA the base is adenine, uracil, guanine, or cytosine.

Nucleus   The subcellular organelle in higher organisms that houses the genetic information.

Oligonucleotide   A short, single-stranded segment of DNA often used as a probe to locate a complementary sequence of DNA or RNA.

Paternity   Identification of the father of a child.

PCR   Abbreviation for *Polymerase chain reaction.*

Pedigree   A diagram that describes family relationships and includes important information about the transmission of one or more diseases that family members share.

Penetrance   A description of the extent to which a disease is expressed within a population; this is measured by calculating the proportion of individuals with a disease-causing genotype who actually manifest the disease.

Peptide   Two or more amino acids covalently linked together.

Phenotype   The observed characteristics of an individual or the physiological makeup that results from the genetic makeup; phenotype is not a foregone conclusion of genotype, because many factors influence which genes are expressed. Even identical twins, who have identical genotypes, can have slightly different phenotypes because of the lifestyle choices they make (compare *Genotype*).

Physical map   A map that gives the locations of identifiable landmarks on DNA, which may be genes or markers such as restriction enzyme cutting sites; distance is measured in base pairs (compare *Genetic linkage map*, in which recombination frequencies are estimated).

Plasmid   A small, circular, extrachromosomal double-stranded DNA molecule capable of reproducing itself within a host cell; plasmids are used as vectors into which foreign genes can be inserted and copied each time the plasmid's DNA is copied.

Polyclonal antibody   An antibody derived from multiple cells rather than from just a single clone of cells, as is a monoclonal antibody; because it is derived from a number of different cells, a polyclonal antibody is actually a mixture of the different monoclonal antibodies produced by each cell.

Polygenic disorders   Disorders resulting from the additive effects of more than one gene; heart disease, cancer, and diabetes are thought to be examples of polygenic disorders.

Polymerase chain reaction (PCR)   An in vitro method of amplifying short DNA segments; this process is sometimes described as molecular photocopying.

Polymorphisms   Naturally occurring variations in a DNA sequence that are useful as genetic markers; technically, a locus is polymorphic when two or more of the alleles at this locus are present in greater than 1% of the population. However, common usage of the term refers simply to multiple alleles (variations, mutations, changes) at a given locus.

Positional cloning   The process of isolating and cloning a disease gene after its approximate physical location has been determined; the function of the gene is often not known at this point.

Postnatal Following birth.

Prenatal Before birth.

Probe A single-stranded segment of DNA tagged in some way, often with radioactivity or fluorescent dye, so that it can be detected when it binds to a DNA segment that contains a sequence complementary to that of the probe; DNA probes are useful in genetic research, in detecting mutations and diseases, and in detecting the presence of infectious organisms in samples of body fluids or in food.

Probiotics Symbiotic microorganisms that can live in the digestive tract of mammals and contribute to the health of the digestive tract (also called friendly microorganisms); examples include strains of *Lactobacillus* and *Bifidobacterium* (lactic acid–producing bacteria) and the yeast *Saccharomyces boulardii.*

Prokaryote An organism that does not have a nucleus, such as a bacterium or blue-green alga; also spelled procaryote (compare *Eukaryote*).

Promoter Segment of DNA within a gene where RNA polymerase binds to begin transcribing the gene, acting as a controlling element in the expression of that gene.

Protein Made up of amino acids; proteins are key molecules produced under the direction of genetic information and responsible for the structure and function of a cell. They carry out the work of the cells and may serve such functions as enzymes, hormones, receptors, transporters, and so on.

Proteome The set of all the proteins coded for in an organism's genetic material.

Proteomics The study of proteomes to identify the proteins within them and the proteins' functions.

Purine A nitrogen-containing, double-ring compound that occurs in nucleic acids; the purines in DNA and RNA are adenine (A) and guanine (G).

Pyrimidine A nitrogen-containing, single-ring compound that occurs in nucleic acids; the pyrimidines in DNA are thymine (T) and cytosine (C); the pyrimidines in RNA are uracil (U) and cytosine (C).

rDNA Abbreviation for *Recombinant DNA.*

Recessive A characteristic that is apparent only when two copies of the gene encoding it are present; in other words, the allele that is not expressed phenotypically (compare *Dominant*).

Recombinant DNA (rDNA) A DNA molecule made by combining DNA from different sources into a single molecule using genetic engineering technology (also called recombinant DNA technology).

Recombinant DNA technology Seminal technology that allowed cutting and pasting of genetic information from different species to create new genetic combinations; this technology gave rise to numerous advances in genetic research.

Recombination Process by which progeny receive genes from both parents to generate a combination different from that of either parent.

Repetitive DNA Nucleotides that exist in multiple copies within the genome, either dispersed throughout the genome or arranged in tandem; their function is unknown, but they have been used to develop DNA typing technology (for identification applications).

Reproductive technology The use of scientific knowledge to assist with conception and gestation of a healthy baby.

Restriction enzymes/endonucleases Known as molecular scissors, proteins that recognize short, specific sequences of DNA and cut the DNA at these sites; restriction enzymes have been essential to the development of recombinant DNA technology and its ability to generate new genetic combinations. They have been useful for systematically generating segments of chromosomes that can be studied, for generating restriction fragment length polymorphisms that can be used to map genes to chromosomal locations, and for developing the technology by which individuals can be identified based on their genetic fingerprints.

Restriction fragment length polymorphism (RFLP)   A variation in DNA sequence (that is, a mutation) such that a restriction enzyme that normally cuts the DNA at this point can no longer do so, thereby generating a different pattern of DNA segments from normal; an RFLP can serve as a useful marker (landmark).

Ribonucleic acid (RNA)   A single-stranded nucleic acid consisting of the bases adenine, guanine, cytosine, and uracil; the sugar ribose; and phosphate. RNA can occur as messenger RNA, transfer RNA, or ribosomal RNA, all of which are involved in protein synthesis.

Ribosomal RNA (rRNA)   A type of RNA directly involved in connecting the appropriate transfer RNA with the codons of messenger RNA during protein synthesis.

Ribosome   The site of protein synthesis, composed of ribosomal RNA and protein.

RNA polymerase   The enzyme that transcribes DNA into RNA.

Sequence tagged site (STS)   A short fragment of DNA, usually consisting of two to five hundred base pairs, that occurs only once in the human genome and whose location and base sequence are known; STSs are useful as markers (landmarks) when constructing the physical map of the human genome. Expressed sequence tags (ESTs) serve the same purpose but are derived from cDNA.

Sequencing   A process whereby the order of the nucleotides in DNA or RNA or the amino acids in protein are determined; DNA sequencing is receiving considerable attention because the base sequence provides valuable information about the composition of a gene, where mutations occur, and the ability to correlate specific mutations with particular effects on function and disease development.

Sex chromosome   In human beings, the X and Y chromosomes that determine the sex of the individual; all the other chromosomes are called autosomes.

Sex-linked   A term describing a trait (marker, gene) that resides on the X or Y chromosome.

Short tandem repeats (STRs)   Short sequences of DNA, usually consisting of two to six base pairs, that are repeated numerous times in head-to-tail fashion; these sequences vary from individual to individual in terms of the number of times the sequence is repeated, forming the basis for identification technology, whereby one individual can be distinguished from any other. Thirteen STR loci form the core of CODIS, the U.S. national database for DNA typing.

Signal transduction   The process by which biochemical messages are communicated between the surface of a cell and its interior.

Single-gene disorder   An inherited condition caused by a mutant allele at a single locus in the DNA; such a trait is monogenic.

Single-stranded DNA   One of the two strands that make up the DNA double helix.

Single nucleotide polymorphism (SNP)   A genetic variation caused by a change in a single DNA nucleotide; most of the variation among individuals results from SNPs. The number of different SNPs in the human population is thought to be in the millions.

SNP   Abbreviation for *Single nucleotide polymorphism.*

Somatic cell   A cell from the body's tissues rather than from the germ line cells (sperm and egg cells).

Southern blot   The process of transferring labeled DNA fragments from a gel matrix to a solid support such as filter paper or a nylon membrane and then detecting the presence of the labeled DNA; this is one part of the process of separating individual DNA fragments from a mixture and probing the various fragments to locate the gene or DNA segment of interest.

Species   A method of classifying organisms; all members of a particular species share common traits that distinguish them from another species.

Spectral karyotype (SKY)   An enhancement to the technique of fluorescent in situ hybridization; by using different colors of fluorescein dyes, each chromosome takes on a different color, such that all 46 human chromosomes can be visualized at one time. This enhancement is particularly useful for observing changes in the normal structure of chromosomes not detectable by traditional methods.

Stem cell   The progenitor cell, an undifferentiated cell that serves as the precursor to specialized cells; human stem cells contain the full set of genetic information and are the subject of much interest for their ability to be developed into virtually any type of cell, including those needed to regenerate an organ for transplantation.

STRs   Abbreviation for *Short tandem repeats.*

Structural genomics   The study of the three-dimensional structure of proteins to better understand their function and to provide considered targets for drug development.

Substitution   A type of mutation in which one base is exchanged (substituted) for another.

Synchotrons   X-ray generators used to study the structure of a protein.

Syndrome   A term used to describe a disease or a condition.

Thymine (T)   A nitrogenous base found in DNA but not in RNA; its complementary base-pairing partner is adenine (A).

Traditional genetics   A term referring to traits inherited in the now-classical Mendelian pattern, which is predictable from the inheritance of chromosomes during gamete formation (compare *Nontraditional genetics*).

Trait   A characteristic associated with a gene that can be quantified or described, such as eye color, flower color, height, intelligence, or the presence of an enzyme.

Transcription   The process by which the information stored in DNA is converted into messenger RNA.

Transcriptomics   A subfield of genetics that involves the large-scale analysis of messenger RNA to determine which genes are expressed, when they are expressed, what controls their expression, and what the transcripts are.

Transfer RNA (tRNA)   A class of RNA involved with matching the amino acid to the messenger RNA template during the synthesis of a protein; the transfer RNA has multiple functional regions, one being the region to which the appropriate amino acid is attached and the other being the anticodon complementary to the codon on the mRNA, which ensures that the appropriate amino acid is inserted at the correct position in the growing protein chain.

Transgenic organisms   Plants or animals in which one or more genes from a different species has been inserted.

Translation   The process by which the information in messenger RNA directs the synthesis of proteins; this process involves mRNA, rRNA, and tRNA.

Translocation   Movement of a segment of a chromosome from its normal site to another chromosome; translocations may be reciprocal, in which segments from two chromosomes exchange positions. There is usually a detrimental effect on health of having the thousands of genes involved change locations.

Transposons   Mobile segments of noncoding DNA that can move from their original position to other locations on the same chromosome or different chromosomes; also called jumping genes. Their function is unknown.

Trisomy   Having an extra copy (three copies total) of a whole chromosome or portion of a chromosome; any chromosome may be involved; results from mistakes made during egg and sperm creation when the members of each chromosome pair fail to separate so that each egg or sperm receives two copies of a chromosome instead of just one. Down syndrome is a medical disorder that results when three copies of chromosome 21 are present in an individual (trisomy 21) or when a partial third copy of chromosome 21 is present.

Tumor suppressor gene   A gene whose product controls cell growth; mutations in tumor suppressor genes can lead to cancer.

Uniparental disomy   A nontraditional mode of inheritance in which one parent has contributed two copies of a chromosome and the other parent has contributed no copy.

Uracil (U)   A nitrogenous base found in RNA but not in DNA; its complementary base-pairing partner is adenine (A).

Variable number of tandem repeats (VNTRs)   Minisatellites of repetitive DNA that vary in the number of repeat units; these polymorphisms are useful in identifying individuals.

Vector   See *Cloning vector.*

Virus   Technically not an organism, consisting only of a protein shell and a nucleic acid genome that may be composed of DNA or RNA; a virus cannot reproduce on its own and must insert its genome into a cell from another organism, commandeer that cell's genetic machinery, and direct it to make more virus particles. Because of this setup, a virus is useful as a vector for carrying foreign DNA and inserting it into the host cell.

VNTR   Abbreviation for *Variable number of tandem repeats.*

X chromosome   The female-associated chromosome in human beings; human females have two such chromosomes.

Xenotransplantation   Organ or tissue donation across species.

Y chromosome   The male-determining chromosome in human beings; human males normally have one Y and one X chromosome.

Yeast artificial chromosome (YAC)   A vector used to clone DNA fragments; YAC can accept up to four hundred base pairs, whereas plasmids typically can only accept one to three hundred base pairs.

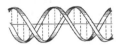

Index